Workout Workbook

By Jennifer Wallner

Today's Goal _____________________   (M) (T) (W) (T) (F) (S) (S)

Muscle Group Focus _______________   Weight ________   Date/Time __________

Stretch ◯   Warm-Up ____

Strength Training

Exercise		Set 1	Set 2	Set 3	Set 4	Set 5	Set 6
	Reps						
	Weight						
	Reps						
	Weight						
	Reps						
	Weight						
	Reps						
	Weight						
	Reps						
	Weight						
	Reps						
	Weight						
	Reps						
	Weight						
	Reps						
	Weight						
	Reps						
	Weight						
	Reps						
	Weight						

Cardio

Exercise	Calories	Distance	Time

Water Intake _________________

Cooldown _________________

Feeling ☆ ☆ ☆ ☆ ☆

Notes

Today's Goal

M T W T F S S

Muscle Group Focus ____________________ Weight ________ Date/Time ________

Stretch ◯   Warm-Up ____________________

Strength Training

Exercise		Set 1	Set 2	Set 3	Set 4	Set 5	Set 6
	Reps						
	Weight						
	Reps						
	Weight						
	Reps						
	Weight						
	Reps						
	Weight						
	Reps						
	Weight						
	Reps						
	Weight						
	Reps						
	Weight						
	Reps						
	Weight						
	Reps						
	Weight						
	Reps						
	Weight						

Cardio

Exercise	Calories	Distance	Time

Water Intake ____________________

Cooldown ____________________

Feeling ☆ ☆ ☆ ☆ ☆

Notes

Today's Goal ____________________   (M) (T) (W) (T) (F) (S) (S)

Muscle Group Focus ________________   Weight ______   Date/Time __________

Stretch ◯   Warm-Up ________________________________

Strength Training

Exercise		Set 1	Set 2	Set 3	Set 4	Set 5	Set 6
	Reps						
	Weight						
	Reps						
	Weight						
	Reps						
	Weight						
	Reps						
	Weight						
	Reps						
	Weight						
	Reps						
	Weight						
	Reps						
	Weight						
	Reps						
	Weight						
	Reps						
	Weight						

Cardio

Exercise	Calories	Distance	Time

Water Intake __________________

Cooldown __________________

Feeling ☆ ☆ ☆ ☆ ☆

Notes

Today's Goal ______________________   Ⓜ Ⓣ Ⓦ Ⓣ Ⓕ ⬤ ⬤

Muscle Group Focus ________________   Weight ______   Date/Time ______

Stretch ◯   Warm-Up ________________________________

Strength Training

Exercise		Set 1	Set 2	Set 3	Set 4	Set 5	Set 6
	Reps						
	Weight						
	Reps						
	Weight						
	Reps						
	Weight						
	Reps						
	Weight						
	Reps						
	Weight						
	Reps						
	Weight						
	Reps						
	Weight						
	Reps						
	Weight						
	Reps						
	Weight						

Cardio

Exercise	Calories	Distance	Time

Water Intake ________________

Cooldown ________________

Feeling ☆ ☆ ☆ ☆ ☆

Notes

Today's Goal ___________________ Ⓜ Ⓣ Ⓦ Ⓣ Ⓕ ⬤S ⬤S

Muscle Group Focus ___________________   Weight ________   Date/Time __________

Stretch ◯   Warm-Up ___________________________________

Strength Training

Exercise		Set 1	Set 2	Set 3	Set 4	Set 5	Set 6
	Reps						
	Weight						
	Reps						
	Weight						
	Reps						
	Weight						
	Reps						
	Weight						
	Reps						
	Weight						
	Reps						
	Weight						
	Reps						
	Weight						
	Reps						
	Weight						
	Reps						
	Weight						

Cardio

Exercise	Calories	Distance	Time

Water Intake ___________________

Cooldown ___________________

Feeling ☆ ☆ ☆ ☆ ☆

Notes

Today's Goal ________________   M T W T F **S** **S**

Muscle Group Focus ________________   Weight ________   Date/Time ________

Stretch ◯   Warm-Up ________________

Strength Training

Exercise		Set 1	Set 2	Set 3	Set 4	Set 5	Set 6
	Reps						
	Weight						
	Reps						
	Weight						
	Reps						
	Weight						
	Reps						
	Weight						
	Reps						
	Weight						
	Reps						
	Weight						
	Reps						
	Weight						
	Reps						
	Weight						
	Reps						
	Weight						

Cardio

Exercise	Calories	Distance	Time

Water Intake ________________

Cooldown ________________

Feeling ☆ ☆ ☆ ☆ ☆

Notes

Today's Goal ___________ Ⓜ Ⓣ Ⓦ Ⓣ Ⓕ Ⓢ Ⓢ

Muscle Group Focus ___________   Weight _______   Date/Time _______

Stretch ◯   Warm-Up ___________

Strength Training

Exercise		Set 1	Set 2	Set 3	Set 4	Set 5	Set 6
	Reps						
	Weight						
	Reps						
	Weight						
	Reps						
	Weight						
	Reps						
	Weight						
	Reps						
	Weight						
	Reps						
	Weight						
	Reps						
	Weight						
	Reps						
	Weight						
	Reps						
	Weight						

Cardio

Exercise	Calories	Distance	Time

Water Intake ___________

Cooldown ___________

Feeling ☆ ☆ ☆ ☆ ☆

Notes

Today's Goal ____________________   (M) (T) (W) (T) (F) (S) (S)

Muscle Group Focus ________________   Weight _______   Date/Time _______

Stretch ◯   Warm-Up ____

Strength Training

Exercise		Set 1	Set 2	Set 3	Set 4	Set 5	Set 6
	Reps						
	Weight						
	Reps						
	Weight						
	Reps						
	Weight						
	Reps						
	Weight						
	Reps						
	Weight						
	Reps						
	Weight						
	Reps						
	Weight						
	Reps						
	Weight						
	Reps						
	Weight						
	Reps						
	Weight						

Cardio

Exercise	Calories	Distance	Time

Water Intake ________________

Cooldown ________________

Feeling ☆ ☆ ☆ ☆ ☆

Notes

Today's Goal ____________________ (M) (T) (W) (T) (F) (S) (S)

Muscle Group Focus ____________________   Weight ________   Date/Time __________

Stretch ◯   Warm-Up ____

Strength Training

Exercise		Set 1	Set 2	Set 3	Set 4	Set 5	Set 6
	Reps						
	Weight						
	Reps						
	Weight						
	Reps						
	Weight						
	Reps						
	Weight						
	Reps						
	Weight						
	Reps						
	Weight						
	Reps						
	Weight						
	Reps						
	Weight						
	Reps						
	Weight						
	Reps						
	Weight						

Cardio

Exercise	Calories	Distance	Time

Water Intake ________________

Cooldown ________________

Feeling ☆ ☆ ☆ ☆ ☆

Notes

Today's Goal ____________________ Ⓜ Ⓣ Ⓦ Ⓣ Ⓕ ⬤S ⬤S

Muscle Group Focus ____________________   Weight ________   Date/Time ________

Stretch ◯   Warm-Up ____________________

Strength Training

Exercise		Set 1	Set 2	Set 3	Set 4	Set 5	Set 6
	Reps						
	Weight						
	Reps						
	Weight						
	Reps						
	Weight						
	Reps						
	Weight						
	Reps						
	Weight						
	Reps						
	Weight						
	Reps						
	Weight						
	Reps						
	Weight						
	Reps						
	Weight						

Cardio

Exercise	Calories	Distance	Time

Water Intake ____________________

Cooldown ____________________

Feeling ☆ ☆ ☆ ☆ ☆

Notes

Today's Goal ________________   (M) (T) (W) (T) (F) (S) (S)

Muscle Group Focus ___________________   Weight _________   Date/Time __________

Stretch ◯   Warm-Up ____

Strength Training

Exercise		Set 1	Set 2	Set 3	Set 4	Set 5	Set 6
	Reps						
	Weight						
	Reps						
	Weight						
	Reps						
	Weight						
	Reps						
	Weight						
	Reps						
	Weight						
	Reps						
	Weight						
	Reps						
	Weight						
	Reps						
	Weight						
	Reps						
	Weight						
	Reps						
	Weight						

Cardio

Exercise	Calories	Distance	Time

Water Intake ___________________

Cooldown ___________________

Feeling ☆ ☆ ☆ ☆ ☆

Notes

Today's Goal ___________________ M T W T F **S** **S**

Muscle Group Focus ___________________   Weight _______   Date/Time _________

Stretch ◯   Warm-Up ___________________

Strength Training

Exercise		Set 1	Set 2	Set 3	Set 4	Set 5	Set 6
	Reps						
	Weight						
	Reps						
	Weight						
	Reps						
	Weight						
	Reps						
	Weight						
	Reps						
	Weight						
	Reps						
	Weight						
	Reps						
	Weight						
	Reps						
	Weight						
	Reps						
	Weight						

Cardio

Exercise	Calories	Distance	Time

Water Intake ___________________

Cooldown ___________________

Feeling ☆ ☆ ☆ ☆ ☆

Notes

Today's Goal

(M) (T) (W) (T) (F) (S) (S)

Muscle Group Focus ______________________ Weight _______ Date/Time __________

Stretch ◯   Warm-Up ____

Strength Training

Exercise		Set 1	Set 2	Set 3	Set 4	Set 5	Set 6
	Reps						
	Weight						
	Reps						
	Weight						
	Reps						
	Weight						
	Reps						
	Weight						
	Reps						
	Weight						
	Reps						
	Weight						
	Reps						
	Weight						
	Reps						
	Weight						
	Reps						
	Weight						
	Reps						
	Weight						

Cardio

Exercise	Calories	Distance	Time

Water Intake _________________

Cooldown _________________

Feeling ☆ ☆ ☆ ☆ ☆

Notes

Today's Goal _______________ Ⓜ Ⓣ Ⓦ Ⓣ Ⓕ ⬤S ⬤S

Muscle Group Focus _______________   Weight _______   Date/Time _______

Stretch ◯   Warm-Up _______________

Strength Training

Exercise		Set 1	Set 2	Set 3	Set 4	Set 5	Set 6
	Reps						
	Weight						
	Reps						
	Weight						
	Reps						
	Weight						
	Reps						
	Weight						
	Reps						
	Weight						
	Reps						
	Weight						
	Reps						
	Weight						
	Reps						
	Weight						
	Reps						
	Weight						
	Reps						
	Weight						

Cardio

Exercise	Calories	Distance	Time

Water Intake _______________

Cooldown _______________

Feeling ☆ ☆ ☆ ☆ ☆

Notes

Today's Goal _______________ M T W T F S S

Muscle Group Focus _______________ Weight _______ Date/Time _______

Stretch ◯   Warm-Up _______________

Strength Training

Exercise		Set 1	Set 2	Set 3	Set 4	Set 5	Set 6
	Reps						
	Weight						
	Reps						
	Weight						
	Reps						
	Weight						
	Reps						
	Weight						
	Reps						
	Weight						
	Reps						
	Weight						
	Reps						
	Weight						
	Reps						
	Weight						
	Reps						
	Weight						

Cardio

Exercise	Calories	Distance	Time

Water Intake _______________

Cooldown _______________

Feeling ☆ ☆ ☆ ☆ ☆

Notes

Today's Goal ____________________   (M) (T) (W) (T) (F) **(S) (S)**

Muscle Group Focus ____________________   Weight ________   Date/Time ________

Stretch ◯   Warm-Up ____________________

Strength Training

Exercise		Set 1	Set 2	Set 3	Set 4	Set 5	Set 6
	Reps						
	Weight						
	Reps						
	Weight						
	Reps						
	Weight						
	Reps						
	Weight						
	Reps						
	Weight						
	Reps						
	Weight						
	Reps						
	Weight						
	Reps						
	Weight						
	Reps						
	Weight						
	Reps						
	Weight						

Cardio

Exercise	Calories	Distance	Time

Water Intake ____________________

Cooldown ____________________

Feeling ☆ ☆ ☆ ☆ ☆

Notes

Today's Goal ______________ Ⓜ Ⓣ Ⓦ Ⓣ Ⓕ ⬤ ⬤

Muscle Group Focus ______________ Weight ______ Date/Time ______

Stretch ◯   Warm-Up ____________________

Strength Training

Exercise		Set 1	Set 2	Set 3	Set 4	Set 5	Set 6
	Reps						
	Weight						
	Reps						
	Weight						
	Reps						
	Weight						
	Reps						
	Weight						
	Reps						
	Weight						
	Reps						
	Weight						
	Reps						
	Weight						
	Reps						
	Weight						
	Reps						
	Weight						
	Reps						
	Weight						

Cardio

Exercise	Calories	Distance	Time

Water Intake ____________

Cooldown ____________

Feeling ☆ ☆ ☆ ☆ ☆

Notes

Today's Goal

M T W T F **S** **S**

Muscle Group Focus ____________________ Weight ________ Date/Time __________

Stretch ◯   Warm-Up ____

Strength Training

Exercise		Set 1	Set 2	Set 3	Set 4	Set 5	Set 6
	Reps						
	Weight						
	Reps						
	Weight						
	Reps						
	Weight						
	Reps						
	Weight						
	Reps						
	Weight						
	Reps						
	Weight						
	Reps						
	Weight						
	Reps						
	Weight						
	Reps						
	Weight						
	Reps						
	Weight						

Cardio

Exercise	Calories	Distance	Time

Water Intake ____________________

Cooldown ____________________

Feeling ☆ ☆ ☆ ☆ ☆

Notes

Today's Goal ____________________   Ⓜ Ⓣ Ⓦ Ⓣ Ⓕ ⬤S ⬤S

Muscle Group Focus ____________________   Weight ________   Date/Time ____________

Stretch ◯   Warm-Up ____

Strength Training

Exercise		Set 1	Set 2	Set 3	Set 4	Set 5	Set 6
	Reps						
	Weight						
	Reps						
	Weight						
	Reps						
	Weight						
	Reps						
	Weight						
	Reps						
	Weight						
	Reps						
	Weight						
	Reps						
	Weight						
	Reps						
	Weight						
	Reps						
	Weight						

Cardio

Exercise	Calories	Distance	Time

Water Intake ____________________

Cooldown ____________________

Feeling ☆ ☆ ☆ ☆ ☆

Notes

Today's Goal ______________________ M T W T F **S** **S**

Muscle Group Focus ____________________   Weight ________   Date/Time __________

Stretch ◯   Warm-Up ___________________________________

Strength Training

Exercise		Set 1	Set 2	Set 3	Set 4	Set 5	Set 6
	Reps						
	Weight						
	Reps						
	Weight						
	Reps						
	Weight						
	Reps						
	Weight						
	Reps						
	Weight						
	Reps						
	Weight						
	Reps						
	Weight						
	Reps						
	Weight						
	Reps						
	Weight						
	Reps						
	Weight						

Cardio

Exercise	Calories	Distance	Time

Water Intake ________________

Cooldown ________________

Feeling ☆ ☆ ☆ ☆ ☆

Notes

Today's Goal ______________________   (M) (T) (W) (T) (F) (S) (S)

Muscle Group Focus ______________   Weight ______   Date/Time __________

Stretch ◯   Warm-Up ___________________________________

Strength Training

Exercise		Set 1	Set 2	Set 3	Set 4	Set 5	Set 6
	Reps						
	Weight						
	Reps						
	Weight						
	Reps						
	Weight						
	Reps						
	Weight						
	Reps						
	Weight						
	Reps						
	Weight						
	Reps						
	Weight						
	Reps						
	Weight						
	Reps						
	Weight						
	Reps						
	Weight						

Cardio

Exercise	Calories	Distance	Time

Water Intake ___________________

Cooldown ___________________

Feeling ☆ ☆ ☆ ☆ ☆

Notes

Today's Goal _______________________   Ⓜ Ⓣ Ⓦ Ⓣ Ⓕ ⬤S ⬤S

Muscle Group Focus _______________   Weight _______   Date/Time _______

Stretch ◯   Warm-Up _______________________________________

Strength Training

Exercise		Set 1	Set 2	Set 3	Set 4	Set 5	Set 6
	Reps						
	Weight						
	Reps						
	Weight						
	Reps						
	Weight						
	Reps						
	Weight						
	Reps						
	Weight						
	Reps						
	Weight						
	Reps						
	Weight						
	Reps						
	Weight						
	Reps						
	Weight						
	Reps						
	Weight						

Cardio

Exercise	Calories	Distance	Time

Water Intake _______________

Cooldown _______________

Feeling ☆ ☆ ☆ ☆ ☆

Notes

Today's Goal ____________________   (M) (T) (W) (T) (F) (S) (S)

Muscle Group Focus ____________________   Weight ________   Date/Time __________

Stretch ◯   Warm-Up ________________________________

Strength Training

Exercise		Set 1	Set 2	Set 3	Set 4	Set 5	Set 6
	Reps						
	Weight						
	Reps						
	Weight						
	Reps						
	Weight						
	Reps						
	Weight						
	Reps						
	Weight						
	Reps						
	Weight						
	Reps						
	Weight						
	Reps						
	Weight						
	Reps						
	Weight						
	Reps						
	Weight						

Cardio

Exercise	Calories	Distance	Time

Water Intake ________________________

Cooldown ________________________

Feeling ☆ ☆ ☆ ☆ ☆

Notes

Today's Goal　___________________　Ⓜ Ⓣ Ⓦ Ⓣ Ⓕ ⬤S ⬤S

Muscle Group Focus　___________________　Weight ________　Date/Time __________

Stretch ◯　　Warm-Up ______________________________

Strength Training

Exercise		Set 1	Set 2	Set 3	Set 4	Set 5	Set 6
	Reps						
	Weight						
	Reps						
	Weight						
	Reps						
	Weight						
	Reps						
	Weight						
	Reps						
	Weight						
	Reps						
	Weight						
	Reps						
	Weight						
	Reps						
	Weight						
	Reps						
	Weight						

Cardio

Exercise	Calories	Distance	Time

Water Intake ______________________

Cooldown ______________________

Feeling ☆ ☆ ☆ ☆ ☆

Notes

Today's Goal

Today's Goal _______________________ (M) (T) (W) (T) (F) (S) (S)

Muscle Group Focus _______________ Weight _______ Date/Time _________

Stretch ◯   Warm-Up _______________________________________

Strength Training

Exercise		Set 1	Set 2	Set 3	Set 4	Set 5	Set 6
	Reps						
	Weight						
	Reps						
	Weight						
	Reps						
	Weight						
	Reps						
	Weight						
	Reps						
	Weight						
	Reps						
	Weight						
	Reps						
	Weight						
	Reps						
	Weight						
	Reps						
	Weight						

Cardio

Exercise	Calories	Distance	Time

Water Intake _______________________

Cooldown _______________________

Feeling ☆ ☆ ☆ ☆ ☆

Notes

Today's Goal ___________________ (M) (T) (W) (T) (F) (S) (S)

Muscle Group Focus ___________________ Weight ________ Date/Time ________

Stretch ◯   Warm-Up ___________________

Strength Training

Exercise		Set 1	Set 2	Set 3	Set 4	Set 5	Set 6
	Reps						
	Weight						
	Reps						
	Weight						
	Reps						
	Weight						
	Reps						
	Weight						
	Reps						
	Weight						
	Reps						
	Weight						
	Reps						
	Weight						
	Reps						
	Weight						
	Reps						
	Weight						
	Reps						
	Weight						

Cardio

Exercise	Calories	Distance	Time

Water Intake ___________________

Cooldown ___________________

Feeling ☆ ☆ ☆ ☆ ☆

Notes

Today's Goal

(M)(T)(W)(T)(F)(**S**)(**S**)

Muscle Group Focus ___________________ Weight _______ Date/Time _______

Stretch ◯ Warm-Up _______________________________

Strength Training

Exercise		Set 1	Set 2	Set 3	Set 4	Set 5	Set 6
	Reps						
	Weight						
	Reps						
	Weight						
	Reps						
	Weight						
	Reps						
	Weight						
	Reps						
	Weight						
	Reps						
	Weight						
	Reps						
	Weight						
	Reps						
	Weight						
	Reps						
	Weight						
	Reps						
	Weight						

Cardio

Exercise	Calories	Distance	Time

Water Intake _______________________

Cooldown _______________________

Feeling ☆ ☆ ☆ ☆ ☆

Notes

Today's Goal _______________   (M) (T) (W) (T) (F) (S) (S)

Muscle Group Focus _______________   Weight _______   Date/Time _______

Stretch ◯   Warm-Up _______________

Strength Training

Exercise		Set 1	Set 2	Set 3	Set 4	Set 5	Set 6
	Reps						
	Weight						
	Reps						
	Weight						
	Reps						
	Weight						
	Reps						
	Weight						
	Reps						
	Weight						
	Reps						
	Weight						
	Reps						
	Weight						
	Reps						
	Weight						
	Reps						
	Weight						

Cardio

Exercise	Calories	Distance	Time
_____			
_____			
_____			

Water Intake _______________

Cooldown _______________

Feeling ☆ ☆ ☆ ☆ ☆

Notes

Today's Goal

Today's Goal _______________________ (M) (T) (W) (T) (F) (S) (S)

Muscle Group Focus _______________ Weight _______ Date/Time _________

Stretch ◯   Warm-Up ____

Strength Training

Exercise		Set 1	Set 2	Set 3	Set 4	Set 5	Set 6
	Reps						
	Weight						
	Reps						
	Weight						
	Reps						
	Weight						
	Reps						
	Weight						
	Reps						
	Weight						
	Reps						
	Weight						
	Reps						
	Weight						
	Reps						
	Weight						
	Reps						
	Weight						
	Reps						
	Weight						

Cardio

Exercise	Calories	Distance	Time

Water Intake _________________

Cooldown _________________

Feeling ☆ ☆ ☆ ☆ ☆

Notes

Today's Goal ____________________   M T W T F **S** **S**

Muscle Group Focus ____________   Weight ______   Date/Time ______

Stretch ◯   Warm-Up ________________________________

Strength Training

Exercise		Set 1	Set 2	Set 3	Set 4	Set 5	Set 6
	Reps						
	Weight						
	Reps						
	Weight						
	Reps						
	Weight						
	Reps						
	Weight						
	Reps						
	Weight						
	Reps						
	Weight						
	Reps						
	Weight						
	Reps						
	Weight						
	Reps						
	Weight						

Cardio

Exercise	Calories	Distance	Time

Water Intake ________________

Cooldown ________________

Feeling ☆ ☆ ☆ ☆ ☆

Notes

Today's Goal ____________________   Ⓜ Ⓣ Ⓦ Ⓣ Ⓕ ⚫S ⚫S

Muscle Group Focus ____________________   Weight ________   Date/Time ________

Stretch ◯   Warm-Up ____________________________________

Strength Training

Exercise		Set 1	Set 2	Set 3	Set 4	Set 5	Set 6
	Reps						
	Weight						
	Reps						
	Weight						
	Reps						
	Weight						
	Reps						
	Weight						
	Reps						
	Weight						
	Reps						
	Weight						
	Reps						
	Weight						
	Reps						
	Weight						
	Reps						
	Weight						
	Reps						
	Weight						

Cardio

Exercise	Calories	Distance	Time

Water Intake ____________________

Cooldown ____________________

Feeling ☆ ☆ ☆ ☆ ☆

Notes

Today's Goal __________________________   (M) (T) (W) (T) (F) (S) (S)

Muscle Group Focus ____________________   Weight ________   Date/Time ___________

Stretch ◯   Warm-Up _______________________________________

Strength Training

Exercise		Set 1	Set 2	Set 3	Set 4	Set 5	Set 6
	Reps						
	Weight						
	Reps						
	Weight						
	Reps						
	Weight						
	Reps						
	Weight						
	Reps						
	Weight						
	Reps						
	Weight						
	Reps						
	Weight						
	Reps						
	Weight						
	Reps						
	Weight						
	Reps						
	Weight						

Cardio

Exercise	Calories	Distance	Time

Water Intake _________________

Cooldown _________________

Feeling ☆ ☆ ☆ ☆ ☆

Notes

Today's Goal ____________________ Ⓜ Ⓣ Ⓦ Ⓣ Ⓕ ⬤S ⬤S

Muscle Group Focus _______________   Weight _______   Date/Time _______

Stretch ◯   Warm-Up ____________________________________

Strength Training

Exercise		Set 1	Set 2	Set 3	Set 4	Set 5	Set 6
	Reps						
	Weight						
	Reps						
	Weight						
	Reps						
	Weight						
	Reps						
	Weight						
	Reps						
	Weight						
	Reps						
	Weight						
	Reps						
	Weight						
	Reps						
	Weight						
	Reps						
	Weight						
	Reps						
	Weight						

Cardio

Exercise	Calories	Distance	Time

Water Intake ____________________

Cooldown ____________________

Feeling ☆ ☆ ☆ ☆ ☆

Notes

Today's Goal _______________ Ⓜ Ⓣ Ⓦ Ⓣ Ⓕ ⬤S ⬤S

Muscle Group Focus _______________   Weight _______   Date/Time _______

Stretch ◯   Warm-Up _______________________________________

Strength Training

Exercise		Set 1	Set 2	Set 3	Set 4	Set 5	Set 6
	Reps						
	Weight						
	Reps						
	Weight						
	Reps						
	Weight						
	Reps						
	Weight						
	Reps						
	Weight						
	Reps						
	Weight						
	Reps						
	Weight						
	Reps						
	Weight						
	Reps						
	Weight						

Cardio

Exercise	Calories	Distance	Time

Water Intake _______________

Cooldown _______________

Feeling ☆ ☆ ☆ ☆ ☆

Notes

Today's Goal

Today's Goal _______________________   (M) (T) (W) (T) (F) (S) (S)

Muscle Group Focus _______________   Weight _______   Date/Time _______

Stretch ◯   Warm-Up _________________________________

Strength Training

Exercise		Set 1	Set 2	Set 3	Set 4	Set 5	Set 6
	Reps						
	Weight						
	Reps						
	Weight						
	Reps						
	Weight						
	Reps						
	Weight						
	Reps						
	Weight						
	Reps						
	Weight						
	Reps						
	Weight						
	Reps						
	Weight						
	Reps						
	Weight						
	Reps						
	Weight						

Cardio

Exercise	Calories	Distance	Time

Water Intake _______________

Cooldown _______________

Feeling ☆ ☆ ☆ ☆ ☆

Notes

Today's Goal ___________________ Ⓜ Ⓣ Ⓦ Ⓣ Ⓕ ⬤S ⬤S

Muscle Group Focus ___________________ Weight _______ Date/Time __________

Stretch ◯   Warm-Up ____

Strength Training

Exercise		Set 1	Set 2	Set 3	Set 4	Set 5	Set 6
	Reps						
	Weight						
	Reps						
	Weight						
	Reps						
	Weight						
	Reps						
	Weight						
	Reps						
	Weight						
	Reps						
	Weight						
	Reps						
	Weight						
	Reps						
	Weight						
	Reps						
	Weight						
	Reps						
	Weight						

Cardio

Exercise	Calories	Distance	Time

Water Intake ___________________

Cooldown ___________________

Feeling ☆ ☆ ☆ ☆ ☆

Notes

Today's Goal ________________________ Ⓜ Ⓣ Ⓦ Ⓣ Ⓕ ⬤S ⬤S

Muscle Group Focus ____________________ Weight ________ Date/Time ____________

Stretch ◯   Warm-Up ____

Strength Training

Exercise		Set 1	Set 2	Set 3	Set 4	Set 5	Set 6
	Reps						
	Weight						
	Reps						
	Weight						
	Reps						
	Weight						
	Reps						
	Weight						
	Reps						
	Weight						
	Reps						
	Weight						
	Reps						
	Weight						
	Reps						
	Weight						
	Reps						
	Weight						
	Reps						
	Weight						

Cardio

Exercise	Calories	Distance	Time

Water Intake ____________________

Cooldown ____________________

Feeling ☆ ☆ ☆ ☆ ☆

Notes

Today's Goal ___________   Ⓜ Ⓣ Ⓦ Ⓣ Ⓕ ⬤S ⬤S

Muscle Group Focus ___________   Weight ______   Date/Time ______

Stretch ◯   Warm-Up ___________

Strength Training

Exercise		Set 1	Set 2	Set 3	Set 4	Set 5	Set 6
	Reps						
	Weight						
	Reps						
	Weight						
	Reps						
	Weight						
	Reps						
	Weight						
	Reps						
	Weight						
	Reps						
	Weight						
	Reps						
	Weight						
	Reps						
	Weight						
	Reps						
	Weight						

Cardio

Exercise	Calories	Distance	Time

Water Intake ___________

Cooldown ___________

Feeling ☆ ☆ ☆ ☆ ☆

Notes

Today's Goal ________________   (M) (T) (W) (T) (F) (S) (S)

Muscle Group Focus ____________________   Weight _______   Date/Time __________

Stretch ◯   Warm-Up ________________________________

Strength Training

Exercise		Set 1	Set 2	Set 3	Set 4	Set 5	Set 6
	Reps						
	Weight						
	Reps						
	Weight						
	Reps						
	Weight						
	Reps						
	Weight						
	Reps						
	Weight						
	Reps						
	Weight						
	Reps						
	Weight						
	Reps						
	Weight						
	Reps						
	Weight						

Cardio

Exercise	Calories	Distance	Time

Water Intake ____________________

Cooldown ____________________

Feeling ☆ ☆ ☆ ☆ ☆

Notes

Today's Goal ______________________   (M) (T) (W) (T) (F) (S) (S)

Muscle Group Focus ____________________   Weight ________   Date/Time __________

Stretch ◯   Warm-Up ________________________________

Strength Training

Exercise		Set 1	Set 2	Set 3	Set 4	Set 5	Set 6
	Reps						
	Weight						
	Reps						
	Weight						
	Reps						
	Weight						
	Reps						
	Weight						
	Reps						
	Weight						
	Reps						
	Weight						
	Reps						
	Weight						
	Reps						
	Weight						
	Reps						
	Weight						
	Reps						
	Weight						

Cardio

Exercise	Calories	Distance	Time

Water Intake ____________________

Cooldown ____________________

Feeling ☆ ☆ ☆ ☆ ☆

Notes

Today's Goal ___________________ Ⓜ Ⓣ Ⓦ Ⓣ Ⓕ Ⓢ Ⓢ

Muscle Group Focus _______________ Weight ______ Date/Time ________

Stretch ◯   Warm-Up ___________________________________

Strength Training

Exercise		Set 1	Set 2	Set 3	Set 4	Set 5	Set 6
	Reps						
	Weight						
	Reps						
	Weight						
	Reps						
	Weight						
	Reps						
	Weight						
	Reps						
	Weight						
	Reps						
	Weight						
	Reps						
	Weight						
	Reps						
	Weight						
	Reps						
	Weight						

Cardio

Exercise	Calories	Distance	Time

Water Intake ___________________

Cooldown ___________________

Feeling ☆ ☆ ☆ ☆ ☆

Notes

Today's Goal ____________________ Ⓜ Ⓣ Ⓦ Ⓣ Ⓕ ⬤S ⬤S

Muscle Group Focus ____________________   Weight ________   Date/Time ________

Stretch ◯   Warm-Up ____________________

Strength Training

Exercise		Set 1	Set 2	Set 3	Set 4	Set 5	Set 6
	Reps						
	Weight						
	Reps						
	Weight						
	Reps						
	Weight						
	Reps						
	Weight						
	Reps						
	Weight						
	Reps						
	Weight						
	Reps						
	Weight						
	Reps						
	Weight						
	Reps						
	Weight						
	Reps						
	Weight						

Cardio

Exercise	Calories	Distance	Time

Water Intake ____________________

Cooldown ____________________

Feeling ☆ ☆ ☆ ☆ ☆

Notes

Today's Goal ___________________ Ⓜ Ⓣ Ⓦ Ⓣ Ⓕ ⬤S ⬤S

Muscle Group Focus ______________   Weight ________   Date/Time __________

Stretch ◯   Warm-Up ________________________________

Strength Training

Exercise		Set 1	Set 2	Set 3	Set 4	Set 5	Set 6
	Reps						
	Weight						
	Reps						
	Weight						
	Reps						
	Weight						
	Reps						
	Weight						
	Reps						
	Weight						
	Reps						
	Weight						
	Reps						
	Weight						
	Reps						
	Weight						
	Reps						
	Weight						
	Reps						
	Weight						

Cardio

Exercise	Calories	Distance	Time

Water Intake __________________

Cooldown __________________

Feeling ☆ ☆ ☆ ☆ ☆

Notes

Today's Goal ____________________   Ⓜ Ⓣ Ⓦ Ⓣ Ⓕ ⬤ ⬤

Muscle Group Focus ____________________   Weight ________   Date/Time ________

Stretch ◯   Warm-Up ____________________

Strength Training

Exercise		Set 1	Set 2	Set 3	Set 4	Set 5	Set 6
	Reps						
	Weight						
	Reps						
	Weight						
	Reps						
	Weight						
	Reps						
	Weight						
	Reps						
	Weight						
	Reps						
	Weight						
	Reps						
	Weight						
	Reps						
	Weight						
	Reps						
	Weight						

Cardio

Exercise	Calories	Distance	Time

Water Intake ____________________

Cooldown ____________________

Feeling ☆ ☆ ☆ ☆ ☆

Notes

Today's Goal ____________________   Ⓜ Ⓣ Ⓦ Ⓣ Ⓕ ⬤S ⬤S

Muscle Group Focus ____________   Weight ______   Date/Time ______

Stretch ◯   Warm-Up ________________________

Strength Training

Exercise		Set 1	Set 2	Set 3	Set 4	Set 5	Set 6
	Reps						
	Weight						
	Reps						
	Weight						
	Reps						
	Weight						
	Reps						
	Weight						
	Reps						
	Weight						
	Reps						
	Weight						
	Reps						
	Weight						
	Reps						
	Weight						
	Reps						
	Weight						
	Reps						
	Weight						

Cardio

Exercise	Calories	Distance	Time

Water Intake ________________

Cooldown ________________

Feeling ☆ ☆ ☆ ☆ ☆

Notes

Today's Goal _______________   (M) (T) (W) (T) (F) (S) (S)

Muscle Group Focus _______________   Weight _______   Date/Time _______

Stretch ◯   Warm-Up _______________

Strength Training

Exercise		Set 1	Set 2	Set 3	Set 4	Set 5	Set 6
	Reps						
	Weight						
	Reps						
	Weight						
	Reps						
	Weight						
	Reps						
	Weight						
	Reps						
	Weight						
	Reps						
	Weight						
	Reps						
	Weight						
	Reps						
	Weight						
	Reps						
	Weight						

Cardio

Exercise	Calories	Distance	Time

Water Intake _______________

Cooldown _______________

Feeling ☆ ☆ ☆ ☆ ☆

Notes

Today's Goal _______________ Ⓜ Ⓣ Ⓦ Ⓣ Ⓕ ⬤S ⬤S

Muscle Group Focus ___________________ Weight ________ Date/Time __________

Stretch ◯   Warm-Up _______________________________

Strength Training

Exercise		Set 1	Set 2	Set 3	Set 4	Set 5	Set 6
	Reps						
	Weight						
	Reps						
	Weight						
	Reps						
	Weight						
	Reps						
	Weight						
	Reps						
	Weight						
	Reps						
	Weight						
	Reps						
	Weight						
	Reps						
	Weight						
	Reps						
	Weight						
	Reps						
	Weight						

Cardio

Exercise	Calories	Distance	Time
________			
________			
________			

Water Intake _______________

Cooldown _______________

Feeling ☆ ☆ ☆ ☆ ☆

Notes

Today's Goal _______________   Ⓜ Ⓣ Ⓦ Ⓣ Ⓕ ⬤S ⬤S

Muscle Group Focus _______________   Weight _______   Date/Time _______

Stretch ◯   Warm-Up _______________

Strength Training

Exercise		Set 1	Set 2	Set 3	Set 4	Set 5	Set 6
	Reps						
	Weight						
	Reps						
	Weight						
	Reps						
	Weight						
	Reps						
	Weight						
	Reps						
	Weight						
	Reps						
	Weight						
	Reps						
	Weight						
	Reps						
	Weight						
	Reps						
	Weight						
	Reps						
	Weight						

Cardio

Exercise	Calories	Distance	Time
_______			
_______			
_______			

Water Intake _______________

Cooldown _______________

Feeling ☆ ☆ ☆ ☆ ☆

Notes

Today's Goal ______________________ Ⓜ Ⓣ Ⓦ Ⓣ Ⓕ ⬤S ⬤S

Muscle Group Focus ______________ Weight ______ Date/Time ______

Stretch ◯   Warm-Up ________________________________

Strength Training

Exercise		Set 1	Set 2	Set 3	Set 4	Set 5	Set 6
	Reps						
	Weight						
	Reps						
	Weight						
	Reps						
	Weight						
	Reps						
	Weight						
	Reps						
	Weight						
	Reps						
	Weight						
	Reps						
	Weight						
	Reps						
	Weight						
	Reps						
	Weight						

Cardio

Exercise	Calories	Distance	Time

Water Intake ______________

Cooldown ______________

Feeling ☆ ☆ ☆ ☆ ☆

Notes

Today's Goal ____________________ Ⓜ Ⓣ Ⓦ Ⓣ Ⓕ ⬤S ⬤S

Muscle Group Focus ____________________   Weight ________   Date/Time __________

Stretch ◯   Warm-Up ____

Strength Training

Exercise		Set 1	Set 2	Set 3	Set 4	Set 5	Set 6
	Reps						
	Weight						
	Reps						
	Weight						
	Reps						
	Weight						
	Reps						
	Weight						
	Reps						
	Weight						
	Reps						
	Weight						
	Reps						
	Weight						
	Reps						
	Weight						
	Reps						
	Weight						
	Reps						
	Weight						

Cardio

Exercise	Calories	Distance	Time

Water Intake ____________________

Cooldown ____________________

Feeling ☆ ☆ ☆ ☆ ☆

Notes

Today's Goal

M T W T F S S

Muscle Group Focus ___________________   Weight _________   Date/Time ___________

Stretch ◯   Warm-Up ____

Strength Training

Exercise		Set 1	Set 2	Set 3	Set 4	Set 5	Set 6
	Reps						
	Weight						
	Reps						
	Weight						
	Reps						
	Weight						
	Reps						
	Weight						
	Reps						
	Weight						
	Reps						
	Weight						
	Reps						
	Weight						
	Reps						
	Weight						
	Reps						
	Weight						
	Reps						
	Weight						

Cardio

Exercise	Calories	Distance	Time

Water Intake _______________________

Cooldown _______________________

Feeling ☆ ☆ ☆ ☆ ☆

Notes

Today's Goal

M T W T F **S** **S**

Muscle Group Focus ___________________   Weight _________   Date/Time ___________

Stretch ◯   Warm-Up ___________________________________

Strength Training

Exercise		Set 1	Set 2	Set 3	Set 4	Set 5	Set 6
	Reps						
	Weight						
	Reps						
	Weight						
	Reps						
	Weight						
	Reps						
	Weight						
	Reps						
	Weight						
	Reps						
	Weight						
	Reps						
	Weight						
	Reps						
	Weight						
	Reps						
	Weight						

Cardio

Exercise	Calories	Distance	Time

Water Intake ___________________

Cooldown ___________________

Feeling ☆ ☆ ☆ ☆ ☆

Notes

Today's Goal _______________ Ⓜ Ⓣ Ⓦ Ⓣ Ⓕ ⬤S ⬤S

Muscle Group Focus _______________ Weight _______ Date/Time _______

Stretch ◯   Warm-Up _______________

Strength Training

Exercise		Set 1	Set 2	Set 3	Set 4	Set 5	Set 6
	Reps						
	Weight						
	Reps						
	Weight						
	Reps						
	Weight						
	Reps						
	Weight						
	Reps						
	Weight						
	Reps						
	Weight						
	Reps						
	Weight						
	Reps						
	Weight						
	Reps						
	Weight						
	Reps						
	Weight						

Cardio

Exercise	Calories	Distance	Time

Water Intake _______________

Cooldown _______________

Feeling ☆ ☆ ☆ ☆ ☆

Notes

Today's Goal   ___________________   Ⓜ Ⓣ Ⓦ Ⓣ Ⓕ ⬤S ⬤S

Muscle Group Focus ___________________   Weight _______   Date/Time __________

Stretch ◯   Warm-Up ____

Strength Training

Exercise			Set 1	Set 2	Set 3	Set 4	Set 5	Set 6
		Reps						
		Weight						
		Reps						
		Weight						
		Reps						
		Weight						
		Reps						
		Weight						
		Reps						
		Weight						
		Reps						
		Weight						
		Reps						
		Weight						
		Reps						
		Weight						
		Reps						
		Weight						

Cardio

Exercise	Calories	Distance	Time

Water Intake ___________________

Cooldown ___________________

Feeling ☆ ☆ ☆ ☆ ☆

Notes

Today's Goal ___________________ Ⓜ Ⓣ Ⓦ Ⓣ Ⓕ ⬤S ⬤S

Muscle Group Focus ___________________ Weight _______ Date/Time _________

Stretch ◯ Warm-Up ___________________________________

Strength Training

Exercise		Set 1	Set 2	Set 3	Set 4	Set 5	Set 6
	Reps						
	Weight						
	Reps						
	Weight						
	Reps						
	Weight						
	Reps						
	Weight						
	Reps						
	Weight						
	Reps						
	Weight						
	Reps						
	Weight						
	Reps						
	Weight						
	Reps						
	Weight						

Cardio

Exercise	Calories	Distance	Time

Water Intake ___________________

Cooldown ___________________

Feeling ☆ ☆ ☆ ☆ ☆

Notes

Today's Goal

(M) (T) (W) (T) (F) (S) (S)

Muscle Group Focus ___________________ Weight ________ Date/Time __________

Stretch ◯ Warm-Up ___________________________________

Strength Training

Exercise		Set 1	Set 2	Set 3	Set 4	Set 5	Set 6
	Reps						
	Weight						
	Reps						
	Weight						
	Reps						
	Weight						
	Reps						
	Weight						
	Reps						
	Weight						
	Reps						
	Weight						
	Reps						
	Weight						
	Reps						
	Weight						
	Reps						
	Weight						

Cardio

Exercise	Calories	Distance	Time

Water Intake ___________________

Cooldown ___________________

Feeling ☆ ☆ ☆ ☆ ☆

Notes

Today's Goal ___________________________   (M) (T) (W) (T) (F) (S) (S)

Muscle Group Focus ___________________   Weight ______   Date/Time ________

Stretch ◯   Warm-Up ____

Strength Training

Exercise		Set 1	Set 2	Set 3	Set 4	Set 5	Set 6
	Reps						
	Weight						
	Reps						
	Weight						
	Reps						
	Weight						
	Reps						
	Weight						
	Reps						
	Weight						
	Reps						
	Weight						
	Reps						
	Weight						
	Reps						
	Weight						
	Reps						
	Weight						

Cardio

Exercise	Calories	Distance	Time

Water Intake ________________

Cooldown ________________

Feeling ☆ ☆ ☆ ☆ ☆

Notes

Today's Goal ___________________________ Ⓜ Ⓣ Ⓦ Ⓣ Ⓕ ⬤S ⬤S

Muscle Group Focus _______________ Weight _______ Date/Time _______

Stretch ◯   Warm-Up _______________________________________

Strength Training

Exercise		Set 1	Set 2	Set 3	Set 4	Set 5	Set 6
	Reps						
	Weight						
	Reps						
	Weight						
	Reps						
	Weight						
	Reps						
	Weight						
	Reps						
	Weight						
	Reps						
	Weight						
	Reps						
	Weight						
	Reps						
	Weight						
	Reps						
	Weight						

Cardio

Exercise	Calories	Distance	Time

Water Intake _______________

Cooldown _______________

Feeling ☆ ☆ ☆ ☆ ☆

Notes

Today's Goal _______________   Ⓜ Ⓣ Ⓦ Ⓣ Ⓕ ⬤S ⬤S

Muscle Group Focus _______________   Weight _______   Date/Time _______

Stretch ◯   Warm-Up _______________

Strength Training

Exercise		Set 1	Set 2	Set 3	Set 4	Set 5	Set 6
	Reps						
	Weight						
	Reps						
	Weight						
	Reps						
	Weight						
	Reps						
	Weight						
	Reps						
	Weight						
	Reps						
	Weight						
	Reps						
	Weight						
	Reps						
	Weight						
	Reps						
	Weight						

Cardio

Exercise	Calories	Distance	Time

Water Intake _______________

Cooldown _______________

Feeling ☆ ☆ ☆ ☆ ☆

Notes

Today's Goal ____________________   M T W T F **S** **S**

Muscle Group Focus ____________________   Weight ________   Date/Time ________

Stretch ◯   Warm-Up ________________________________

Strength Training

Exercise		Set 1	Set 2	Set 3	Set 4	Set 5	Set 6
	Reps						
	Weight						
	Reps						
	Weight						
	Reps						
	Weight						
	Reps						
	Weight						
	Reps						
	Weight						
	Reps						
	Weight						
	Reps						
	Weight						
	Reps						
	Weight						
	Reps						
	Weight						
	Reps						
	Weight						

Cardio

Exercise	Calories	Distance	Time

Water Intake ________________

Cooldown ________________

Feeling ☆ ☆ ☆ ☆ ☆

Notes

Today's Goal _______________________   Ⓜ Ⓣ Ⓦ Ⓣ Ⓕ ⬤ ⬤

Muscle Group Focus _______________   Weight _______   Date/Time _______

Stretch ◯   Warm-Up _______________________________

Strength Training

Exercise		Set 1	Set 2	Set 3	Set 4	Set 5	Set 6
	Reps						
	Weight						
	Reps						
	Weight						
	Reps						
	Weight						
	Reps						
	Weight						
	Reps						
	Weight						
	Reps						
	Weight						
	Reps						
	Weight						
	Reps						
	Weight						
	Reps						
	Weight						

Cardio

Exercise	Calories	Distance	Time

Water Intake _______________

Cooldown _______________

Feeling ☆ ☆ ☆ ☆ ☆

Notes

Today's Goal ______________________ (M) (T) (W) (T) (F) (S) (S)

Muscle Group Focus ________________   Weight ______   Date/Time ________

Stretch ◯   Warm-Up ______________________________

Strength Training

Exercise		Set 1	Set 2	Set 3	Set 4	Set 5	Set 6
	Reps						
	Weight						
	Reps						
	Weight						
	Reps						
	Weight						
	Reps						
	Weight						
	Reps						
	Weight						
	Reps						
	Weight						
	Reps						
	Weight						
	Reps						
	Weight						
	Reps						
	Weight						
	Reps						
	Weight						

Cardio

Exercise	Calories	Distance	Time

Water Intake ________________

Cooldown ________________

Feeling ☆ ☆ ☆ ☆ ☆

Notes

Today's Goal ___________________ Ⓜ Ⓣ Ⓦ Ⓣ Ⓕ ⬤S ⬤S

Muscle Group Focus ___________________ Weight _______ Date/Time _______

Stretch ◯   Warm-Up ___________________

Strength Training

Exercise		Set 1	Set 2	Set 3	Set 4	Set 5	Set 6
	Reps						
	Weight						
	Reps						
	Weight						
	Reps						
	Weight						
	Reps						
	Weight						
	Reps						
	Weight						
	Reps						
	Weight						
	Reps						
	Weight						
	Reps						
	Weight						
	Reps						
	Weight						

Cardio

Exercise	Calories	Distance	Time

Water Intake ___________________

Cooldown ___________________

Feeling ☆ ☆ ☆ ☆ ☆

Notes

Today's Goal ______________________   (M) (T) (W) (T) (F) (S) (S)

Muscle Group Focus ______________   Weight ________   Date/Time __________

Stretch ◯   Warm-Up ______________________________

Strength Training

Exercise		Set 1	Set 2	Set 3	Set 4	Set 5	Set 6
	Reps						
	Weight						
	Reps						
	Weight						
	Reps						
	Weight						
	Reps						
	Weight						
	Reps						
	Weight						
	Reps						
	Weight						
	Reps						
	Weight						
	Reps						
	Weight						
	Reps						
	Weight						

Cardio

Exercise	Calories	Distance	Time

Water Intake ______________

Cooldown ______________

Feeling ☆ ☆ ☆ ☆ ☆

Notes

Today's Goal _______________   Ⓜ Ⓣ Ⓦ Ⓣ Ⓕ ⬤ ⬤

Muscle Group Focus _______________   Weight _______   Date/Time _______

Stretch ◯   Warm-Up _______________________________

Strength Training

Exercise		Set 1	Set 2	Set 3	Set 4	Set 5	Set 6
	Reps						
	Weight						
	Reps						
	Weight						
	Reps						
	Weight						
	Reps						
	Weight						
	Reps						
	Weight						
	Reps						
	Weight						
	Reps						
	Weight						
	Reps						
	Weight						
	Reps						
	Weight						
	Reps						
	Weight						

Cardio

Exercise	Calories	Distance	Time

Water Intake _______________

Cooldown _______________

Feeling ☆ ☆ ☆ ☆ ☆

Notes

Today's Goal ____________________   (M) (T) (W) (T) (F) (S) (S)

Muscle Group Focus ____________________   Weight ________   Date/Time __________

Stretch ◯   Warm-Up ____________________________________

Strength Training

Exercise		Set 1	Set 2	Set 3	Set 4	Set 5	Set 6
	Reps						
	Weight						
	Reps						
	Weight						
	Reps						
	Weight						
	Reps						
	Weight						
	Reps						
	Weight						
	Reps						
	Weight						
	Reps						
	Weight						
	Reps						
	Weight						
	Reps						
	Weight						

Cardio

Exercise	Calories	Distance	Time

Water Intake ____________________

Cooldown ____________________

Feeling ☆ ☆ ☆ ☆ ☆

Notes

Today's Goal ____________________   M T W T F **S** **S**

Muscle Group Focus ________________   Weight ________   Date/Time __________

Stretch ◯   Warm-Up ____

Strength Training

Exercise		Set 1	Set 2	Set 3	Set 4	Set 5	Set 6
	Reps						
	Weight						
	Reps						
	Weight						
	Reps						
	Weight						
	Reps						
	Weight						
	Reps						
	Weight						
	Reps						
	Weight						
	Reps						
	Weight						
	Reps						
	Weight						
	Reps						
	Weight						
	Reps						
	Weight						

Cardio

Exercise	Calories	Distance	Time

Water Intake ________________

Cooldown ________________

Feeling ☆ ☆ ☆ ☆ ☆

Notes

Today's Goal ____________________   Ⓜ Ⓣ Ⓦ Ⓣ Ⓕ ⬤S ⬤S

Muscle Group Focus ____________________   Weight ________   Date/Time ________

Stretch ◯   Warm-Up ____________________

Strength Training

Exercise			Set 1	Set 2	Set 3	Set 4	Set 5	Set 6
	Reps							
	Weight							
	Reps							
	Weight							
	Reps							
	Weight							
	Reps							
	Weight							
	Reps							
	Weight							
	Reps							
	Weight							
	Reps							
	Weight							
	Reps							
	Weight							
	Reps							
	Weight							
	Reps							
	Weight							

Cardio

Exercise	Calories	Distance	Time

Water Intake ____________________

Cooldown ____________________

Feeling ☆ ☆ ☆ ☆ ☆

Notes

Today's Goal

_______________________ Ⓜ Ⓣ Ⓦ Ⓣ Ⓕ ⬤S ⬤S

Muscle Group Focus _______________ Weight _______ Date/Time _______

Stretch ◯   Warm-Up ___________________________

Strength Training

Exercise		Set 1	Set 2	Set 3	Set 4	Set 5	Set 6
	Reps						
	Weight						
	Reps						
	Weight						
	Reps						
	Weight						
	Reps						
	Weight						
	Reps						
	Weight						
	Reps						
	Weight						
	Reps						
	Weight						
	Reps						
	Weight						
	Reps						
	Weight						
	Reps						
	Weight						

Cardio

Exercise	Calories	Distance	Time

Water Intake ___________________________

Cooldown ___________________________

Feeling ☆ ☆ ☆ ☆ ☆

Notes

Today's Goal _______________ Ⓜ Ⓣ Ⓦ Ⓣ Ⓕ ⬤S ⬤S

Muscle Group Focus _______________ Weight _______ Date/Time _______

Stretch ◯   Warm-Up _______________

Strength Training

Exercise		Set 1	Set 2	Set 3	Set 4	Set 5	Set 6
	Reps						
	Weight						
	Reps						
	Weight						
	Reps						
	Weight						
	Reps						
	Weight						
	Reps						
	Weight						
	Reps						
	Weight						
	Reps						
	Weight						
	Reps						
	Weight						
	Reps						
	Weight						

Cardio

Exercise	Calories	Distance	Time

Water Intake _______________

Cooldown _______________

Feeling ☆ ☆ ☆ ☆ ☆

Notes

Today's Goal _______________________   (M) (T) (W) (T) (F) (S) (S)

Muscle Group Focus _______________________   Weight _________   Date/Time _________

Stretch ◯   Warm-Up _______________________

Strength Training

Exercise		Set 1	Set 2	Set 3	Set 4	Set 5	Set 6
	Reps						
	Weight						
	Reps						
	Weight						
	Reps						
	Weight						
	Reps						
	Weight						
	Reps						
	Weight						
	Reps						
	Weight						
	Reps						
	Weight						
	Reps						
	Weight						
	Reps						
	Weight						
	Reps						
	Weight						

Cardio

Exercise	Calories	Distance	Time

Water Intake _______________________

Cooldown _______________________

Feeling ☆ ☆ ☆ ☆ ☆

Notes

Today's Goal ___________________ (M) (T) (W) (T) (F) (S) (S)

Muscle Group Focus ___________________ Weight _______ Date/Time _______

Stretch ◯   Warm-Up _________________________________

Strength Training

Exercise		Set 1	Set 2	Set 3	Set 4	Set 5	Set 6
	Reps						
	Weight						
	Reps						
	Weight						
	Reps						
	Weight						
	Reps						
	Weight						
	Reps						
	Weight						
	Reps						
	Weight						
	Reps						
	Weight						
	Reps						
	Weight						
	Reps						
	Weight						

Cardio

Exercise	Calories	Distance	Time

Water Intake _______

Cooldown _______

Feeling ☆ ☆ ☆ ☆ ☆

Notes

Today's Goal ___________________   Ⓜ Ⓣ Ⓦ Ⓣ Ⓕ ⬤ ⬤

Muscle Group Focus ________________   Weight ________   Date/Time __________

Stretch ◯   Warm-Up ________________________________

Strength Training

Exercise		Set 1	Set 2	Set 3	Set 4	Set 5	Set 6
	Reps						
	Weight						
	Reps						
	Weight						
	Reps						
	Weight						
	Reps						
	Weight						
	Reps						
	Weight						
	Reps						
	Weight						
	Reps						
	Weight						
	Reps						
	Weight						
	Reps						
	Weight						

Cardio

Exercise	Calories	Distance	Time

Water Intake ______________________

Cooldown ______________________

Feeling ☆ ☆ ☆ ☆ ☆

Notes

Today's Goal _______________ Ⓜ Ⓣ Ⓦ Ⓣ Ⓕ ⬤S ⬤S

Muscle Group Focus _______________ Weight ______ Date/Time ______

Stretch ◯   Warm-Up _______________

Strength Training

Exercise		Set 1	Set 2	Set 3	Set 4	Set 5	Set 6
	Reps						
	Weight						
	Reps						
	Weight						
	Reps						
	Weight						
	Reps						
	Weight						
	Reps						
	Weight						
	Reps						
	Weight						
	Reps						
	Weight						
	Reps						
	Weight						
	Reps						
	Weight						

Cardio

Exercise	Calories	Distance	Time

Water Intake _______________

Cooldown _______________

Feeling ☆ ☆ ☆ ☆ ☆

Notes

Today's Goal ____________________   (M) (T) (W) (T) (F) **(S)** **(S)**

Muscle Group Focus ____________________   Weight ________   Date/Time __________

Stretch ◯   Warm-Up ____

Strength Training

Exercise		Set 1	Set 2	Set 3	Set 4	Set 5	Set 6
	Reps						
	Weight						
	Reps						
	Weight						
	Reps						
	Weight						
	Reps						
	Weight						
	Reps						
	Weight						
	Reps						
	Weight						
	Reps						
	Weight						
	Reps						
	Weight						
	Reps						
	Weight						
	Reps						
	Weight						

Cardio

Exercise	Calories	Distance	Time

Water Intake ____________________

Cooldown ____________________

Feeling ☆ ☆ ☆ ☆ ☆

Notes

____

Today's Goal ___________________ Ⓜ Ⓣ Ⓦ Ⓣ Ⓕ ⬤ ⬤

Muscle Group Focus ______________   Weight ______   Date/Time ______

Stretch ◯   Warm-Up ______________________________

Strength Training

Exercise		Set 1	Set 2	Set 3	Set 4	Set 5	Set 6
	Reps						
	Weight						
	Reps						
	Weight						
	Reps						
	Weight						
	Reps						
	Weight						
	Reps						
	Weight						
	Reps						
	Weight						
	Reps						
	Weight						
	Reps						
	Weight						
	Reps						
	Weight						

Cardio

Exercise	Calories	Distance	Time

Water Intake ______________

Cooldown ______________

Feeling ☆ ☆ ☆ ☆ ☆

Notes

Today's Goal _____________ Ⓜ Ⓣ Ⓦ Ⓣ Ⓕ ⓢ ⓢ

Muscle Group Focus _____________ Weight _______ Date/Time _______

Stretch ◯   Warm-Up _____________

Strength Training

Exercise		Set 1	Set 2	Set 3	Set 4	Set 5	Set 6
	Reps						
	Weight						
	Reps						
	Weight						
	Reps						
	Weight						
	Reps						
	Weight						
	Reps						
	Weight						
	Reps						
	Weight						
	Reps						
	Weight						
	Reps						
	Weight						
	Reps						
	Weight						

Cardio

Exercise	Calories	Distance	Time

Water Intake _____________

Cooldown _____________

Feeling ☆ ☆ ☆ ☆ ☆

Notes

Today's Goal

M T W T F **S** **S**

Muscle Group Focus ____________________ Weight ________ Date/Time ____________

Stretch ◯   Warm-Up ____

Strength Training

Exercise		Set 1	Set 2	Set 3	Set 4	Set 5	Set 6
	Reps						
	Weight						
	Reps						
	Weight						
	Reps						
	Weight						
	Reps						
	Weight						
	Reps						
	Weight						
	Reps						
	Weight						
	Reps						
	Weight						
	Reps						
	Weight						
	Reps						
	Weight						

Cardio

Exercise	Calories	Distance	Time

Water Intake ____________________

Cooldown ____________________

Feeling ☆ ☆ ☆ ☆ ☆

Notes

Today's Goal ___________________________   Ⓜ Ⓣ Ⓦ Ⓣ Ⓕ ⑤ ⑤

Muscle Group Focus ___________________   Weight _______   Date/Time _________

Stretch ◯   Warm-Up _______________________________________

Strength Training

Exercise		Set 1	Set 2	Set 3	Set 4	Set 5	Set 6
	Reps						
	Weight						
	Reps						
	Weight						
	Reps						
	Weight						
	Reps						
	Weight						
	Reps						
	Weight						
	Reps						
	Weight						
	Reps						
	Weight						
	Reps						
	Weight						
	Reps						
	Weight						
	Reps						
	Weight						

Cardio

Exercise	Calories	Distance	Time

Water Intake _______________________

Cooldown _______________________

Feeling ☆ ☆ ☆ ☆ ☆

Notes

Today's Goal ______________________   (M) (T) (W) (T) (F) (S) (S)

Muscle Group Focus ________________   Weight ________   Date/Time __________

Stretch ◯   Warm-Up ____

Strength Training

Exercise		Set 1	Set 2	Set 3	Set 4	Set 5	Set 6
	Reps						
	Weight						
	Reps						
	Weight						
	Reps						
	Weight						
	Reps						
	Weight						
	Reps						
	Weight						
	Reps						
	Weight						
	Reps						
	Weight						
	Reps						
	Weight						
	Reps						
	Weight						
	Reps						
	Weight						

Cardio

Exercise	Calories	Distance	Time

Water Intake ___________________

Cooldown ___________________

Feeling ☆ ☆ ☆ ☆ ☆

Notes

Today's Goal ______________________ Ⓜ Ⓣ Ⓦ Ⓣ Ⓕ ⬤S ⬤S

Muscle Group Focus ______________________ Weight _______ Date/Time _______

Stretch ◯ Warm-Up ________________________________

Strength Training

Exercise		Set 1	Set 2	Set 3	Set 4	Set 5	Set 6
	Reps						
	Weight						
	Reps						
	Weight						
	Reps						
	Weight						
	Reps						
	Weight						
	Reps						
	Weight						
	Reps						
	Weight						
	Reps						
	Weight						
	Reps						
	Weight						
	Reps						
	Weight						
	Reps						
	Weight						

Cardio

Exercise	Calories	Distance	Time

Water Intake ________________

Cooldown ________________

Feeling ☆ ☆ ☆ ☆ ☆

Notes

Today's Goal

_________________________   (M) (T) (W) (T) (F) (S) (S)

Muscle Group Focus _______________   Weight _______   Date/Time _______

Stretch ◯   Warm-Up _________________________________

Strength Training

Exercise		Set 1	Set 2	Set 3	Set 4	Set 5	Set 6
	Reps						
	Weight						
	Reps						
	Weight						
	Reps						
	Weight						
	Reps						
	Weight						
	Reps						
	Weight						
	Reps						
	Weight						
	Reps						
	Weight						
	Reps						
	Weight						
	Reps						
	Weight						
	Reps						
	Weight						

Cardio

Exercise	Calories	Distance	Time

Water Intake _________________

Cooldown _________________

Feeling ☆ ☆ ☆ ☆ ☆

Notes

Today's Goal ___________________   (M) (T) (W) (T) (F) (S) (S)

Muscle Group Focus ___________________   Weight ________   Date/Time __________

Stretch ◯   Warm-Up ___________________

Strength Training

Exercise		Set 1	Set 2	Set 3	Set 4	Set 5	Set 6
	Reps						
	Weight						
	Reps						
	Weight						
	Reps						
	Weight						
	Reps						
	Weight						
	Reps						
	Weight						
	Reps						
	Weight						
	Reps						
	Weight						
	Reps						
	Weight						
	Reps						
	Weight						
	Reps						
	Weight						

Cardio

Exercise	Calories	Distance	Time

Water Intake ___________________

Cooldown ___________________

Feeling ☆ ☆ ☆ ☆ ☆

Notes

Today's Goal

(M) (T) (W) (T) (F) (**S**) (**S**)

Muscle Group Focus ______________   Weight ________   Date/Time ________

Stretch ◯   Warm-Up ______________________________________

Strength Training

Exercise		Set 1	Set 2	Set 3	Set 4	Set 5	Set 6
	Reps						
	Weight						
	Reps						
	Weight						
	Reps						
	Weight						
	Reps						
	Weight						
	Reps						
	Weight						
	Reps						
	Weight						
	Reps						
	Weight						
	Reps						
	Weight						
	Reps						
	Weight						
	Reps						
	Weight						

Cardio

Exercise	Calories	Distance	Time

Water Intake ______________

Cooldown ______________

Feeling ☆ ☆ ☆ ☆ ☆

Notes

Today's Goal ___________ Ⓜ Ⓣ Ⓦ Ⓣ Ⓕ ⬤S ⬤S

Muscle Group Focus ___________   Weight ______   Date/Time ______

Stretch ◯   Warm-Up ___________

Strength Training

Exercise		Set 1	Set 2	Set 3	Set 4	Set 5	Set 6
	Reps						
	Weight						
	Reps						
	Weight						
	Reps						
	Weight						
	Reps						
	Weight						
	Reps						
	Weight						
	Reps						
	Weight						
	Reps						
	Weight						
	Reps						
	Weight						
	Reps						
	Weight						

Cardio

Exercise	Calories	Distance	Time

Water Intake ___________

Cooldown ___________

Feeling ☆ ☆ ☆ ☆ ☆

Notes

Today's Goal

Today's Goal _______________________   (M) (T) (W) (T) (F) (S) (S)

Muscle Group Focus _______________   Weight ______   Date/Time ______

Stretch ◯   Warm-Up _______________________________

Strength Training

Exercise		Set 1	Set 2	Set 3	Set 4	Set 5	Set 6
	Reps						
	Weight						
	Reps						
	Weight						
	Reps						
	Weight						
	Reps						
	Weight						
	Reps						
	Weight						
	Reps						
	Weight						
	Reps						
	Weight						
	Reps						
	Weight						
	Reps						
	Weight						
	Reps						
	Weight						

Cardio

Exercise	Calories	Distance	Time

Water Intake _______________________

Cooldown _______________________

Feeling ☆ ☆ ☆ ☆ ☆

Notes

Today's Goal ___________________ Ⓜ Ⓣ Ⓦ Ⓣ Ⓕ Ⓢ Ⓢ

Muscle Group Focus ___________________   Weight _______   Date/Time _______

Stretch ○   Warm-Up ___________________

Strength Training

Exercise		Set 1	Set 2	Set 3	Set 4	Set 5	Set 6
	Reps						
	Weight						
	Reps						
	Weight						
	Reps						
	Weight						
	Reps						
	Weight						
	Reps						
	Weight						
	Reps						
	Weight						
	Reps						
	Weight						
	Reps						
	Weight						
	Reps						
	Weight						

Cardio

Exercise	Calories	Distance	Time

Water Intake ___________________

Cooldown ___________________

Feeling ☆ ☆ ☆ ☆ ☆

Notes

Today's Goal

Today's Goal ____________________   (M) (T) (W) (T) (F) (S) (S)

Muscle Group Focus ____________________   Weight ________   Date/Time ________

Stretch ○   Warm-Up ____________________

Strength Training

Exercise		Set 1	Set 2	Set 3	Set 4	Set 5	Set 6
	Reps						
	Weight						
	Reps						
	Weight						
	Reps						
	Weight						
	Reps						
	Weight						
	Reps						
	Weight						
	Reps						
	Weight						
	Reps						
	Weight						
	Reps						
	Weight						
	Reps						
	Weight						
	Reps						
	Weight						

Cardio

Exercise	Calories	Distance	Time

Water Intake ____________________

Cooldown ____________________

Feeling ☆ ☆ ☆ ☆ ☆

Notes

Today's Goal ______________________   (M) (T) (W) (T) (F) (S) (S)

Muscle Group Focus ________________   Weight ________   Date/Time ________

Stretch ◯   Warm-Up ________________________________

Strength Training

Exercise		Set 1	Set 2	Set 3	Set 4	Set 5	Set 6
	Reps						
	Weight						
	Reps						
	Weight						
	Reps						
	Weight						
	Reps						
	Weight						
	Reps						
	Weight						
	Reps						
	Weight						
	Reps						
	Weight						
	Reps						
	Weight						
	Reps						
	Weight						
	Reps						
	Weight						

Cardio

Exercise	Calories	Distance	Time

Water Intake ________________

Cooldown ________________

Feeling ☆ ☆ ☆ ☆ ☆

Notes

Today's Goal ________________ (M) (T) (W) (T) (F) (S) (S)

Muscle Group Focus ________________   Weight ______   Date/Time ________

Stretch ◯   Warm-Up ________________________________

Strength Training

Exercise		Set 1	Set 2	Set 3	Set 4	Set 5	Set 6
	Reps						
	Weight						
	Reps						
	Weight						
	Reps						
	Weight						
	Reps						
	Weight						
	Reps						
	Weight						
	Reps						
	Weight						
	Reps						
	Weight						
	Reps						
	Weight						
	Reps						
	Weight						
	Reps						
	Weight						

Cardio

Exercise	Calories	Distance	Time

Water Intake ________________

Cooldown ________________

Feeling ☆ ☆ ☆ ☆ ☆

Notes

Today's Goal _______________   M T W T F **S** **S**

Muscle Group Focus _______________   Weight _______   Date/Time _______

Stretch ◯   Warm-Up _______________

Strength Training

Exercise		Set 1	Set 2	Set 3	Set 4	Set 5	Set 6
	Reps						
	Weight						
	Reps						
	Weight						
	Reps						
	Weight						
	Reps						
	Weight						
	Reps						
	Weight						
	Reps						
	Weight						
	Reps						
	Weight						
	Reps						
	Weight						
	Reps						
	Weight						

Cardio

Exercise	Calories	Distance	Time

Water Intake _______________

Cooldown _______________

Feeling ☆ ☆ ☆ ☆ ☆

Notes

Today's Goal   ________________   (M) (T) (W) (T) (F) (S) (S)

Muscle Group Focus ________________   Weight ________   Date/Time ________

Stretch ◯   Warm-Up ________________________________

Strength Training

Exercise		Set 1	Set 2	Set 3	Set 4	Set 5	Set 6
	Reps						
	Weight						
	Reps						
	Weight						
	Reps						
	Weight						
	Reps						
	Weight						
	Reps						
	Weight						
	Reps						
	Weight						
	Reps						
	Weight						
	Reps						
	Weight						
	Reps						
	Weight						
	Reps						
	Weight						

Cardio

Exercise	Calories	Distance	Time

Water Intake ________________

Cooldown ________________

Feeling ☆ ☆ ☆ ☆ ☆

Notes

Today's Goal _______________   Ⓜ Ⓣ Ⓦ Ⓣ Ⓕ ● ●

Muscle Group Focus _______________   Weight ________   Date/Time __________

Stretch ◯   Warm-Up _______________________________

Strength Training

Exercise		Set 1	Set 2	Set 3	Set 4	Set 5	Set 6
	Reps						
	Weight						
	Reps						
	Weight						
	Reps						
	Weight						
	Reps						
	Weight						
	Reps						
	Weight						
	Reps						
	Weight						
	Reps						
	Weight						
	Reps						
	Weight						
	Reps						
	Weight						

Cardio

Exercise	Calories	Distance	Time

Water Intake _______________

Cooldown _______________

Feeling ☆ ☆ ☆ ☆ ☆

Notes

Today's Goal ____________________ Ⓜ Ⓣ Ⓦ Ⓣ Ⓕ ⬤S ⬤S

Muscle Group Focus ____________________   Weight ________   Date/Time __________

Stretch ◯   Warm-Up ____________________________________

Strength Training

Exercise		Set 1	Set 2	Set 3	Set 4	Set 5	Set 6
	Reps						
	Weight						
	Reps						
	Weight						
	Reps						
	Weight						
	Reps						
	Weight						
	Reps						
	Weight						
	Reps						
	Weight						
	Reps						
	Weight						
	Reps						
	Weight						
	Reps						
	Weight						
	Reps						
	Weight						

Cardio

Exercise	Calories	Distance	Time

Water Intake ____________________

Cooldown ____________________

Feeling ☆ ☆ ☆ ☆ ☆

Notes

Today's Goal ____________________   (M) (T) (W) (T) (F) (S) (S)

Muscle Group Focus ____________________   Weight ________   Date/Time __________

Stretch ◯   Warm-Up ____________________________

Strength Training

Exercise		Set 1	Set 2	Set 3	Set 4	Set 5	Set 6
	Reps						
	Weight						
	Reps						
	Weight						
	Reps						
	Weight						
	Reps						
	Weight						
	Reps						
	Weight						
	Reps						
	Weight						
	Reps						
	Weight						
	Reps						
	Weight						
	Reps						
	Weight						

Cardio

Exercise	Calories	Distance	Time

Water Intake ____________________

Cooldown ____________________

Feeling ☆ ☆ ☆ ☆ ☆

Notes

Today's Goal   ___________________   (M) (T) (W) (T) (F) **(S)** **(S)**

Muscle Group Focus ___________________   Weight _______   Date/Time __________

Stretch ◯   Warm-Up ____

Strength Training

Exercise		Set 1	Set 2	Set 3	Set 4	Set 5	Set 6
	Reps						
	Weight						
	Reps						
	Weight						
	Reps						
	Weight						
	Reps						
	Weight						
	Reps						
	Weight						
	Reps						
	Weight						
	Reps						
	Weight						
	Reps						
	Weight						
	Reps						
	Weight						
	Reps						
	Weight						

Cardio

Exercise	Calories	Distance	Time

Water Intake ___________________

Cooldown ___________________

Feeling ☆ ☆ ☆ ☆ ☆

Notes

Today's Goal ________________   (M) (T) (W) (T) (F) (S) (S)

Muscle Group Focus ________________   Weight ______   Date/Time ______

Stretch ◯   Warm-Up ________________________________

Strength Training

Exercise		Set 1	Set 2	Set 3	Set 4	Set 5	Set 6
	Reps						
	Weight						
	Reps						
	Weight						
	Reps						
	Weight						
	Reps						
	Weight						
	Reps						
	Weight						
	Reps						
	Weight						
	Reps						
	Weight						
	Reps						
	Weight						
	Reps						
	Weight						
	Reps						
	Weight						

Cardio

Exercise	Calories	Distance	Time

Water Intake ________________

Cooldown ________________

Feeling ☆ ☆ ☆ ☆ ☆

Notes

Today's Goal _______________   Ⓜ Ⓣ Ⓦ Ⓣ Ⓕ ⬤S ⬤S

Muscle Group Focus _____________   Weight _______   Date/Time _______

Stretch ◯   Warm-Up _______________________________________

Strength Training

Exercise		Set 1	Set 2	Set 3	Set 4	Set 5	Set 6
	Reps						
	Weight						
	Reps						
	Weight						
	Reps						
	Weight						
	Reps						
	Weight						
	Reps						
	Weight						
	Reps						
	Weight						
	Reps						
	Weight						
	Reps						
	Weight						
	Reps						
	Weight						
	Reps						
	Weight						

Cardio

Exercise	Calories	Distance	Time

Water Intake _______________

Cooldown _______________

Feeling ☆ ☆ ☆ ☆ ☆

Notes

Today's Goal _______________________ Ⓜ Ⓣ Ⓦ Ⓣ Ⓕ ⬤S ⬤S

Muscle Group Focus _______________ Weight ______ Date/Time ______

Stretch ◯ Warm-Up _______________________________

Strength Training

Exercise		Set 1	Set 2	Set 3	Set 4	Set 5	Set 6
	Reps						
	Weight						
	Reps						
	Weight						
	Reps						
	Weight						
	Reps						
	Weight						
	Reps						
	Weight						
	Reps						
	Weight						
	Reps						
	Weight						
	Reps						
	Weight						
	Reps						
	Weight						
	Reps						
	Weight						

Cardio

Exercise	Calories	Distance	Time

Water Intake _______________

Cooldown _______________

Feeling ☆ ☆ ☆ ☆ ☆

Notes

Today's Goal ______________________   (M) (T) (W) (T) (F) (S) (S)

Muscle Group Focus ________________   Weight _______   Date/Time _________

Stretch ◯   Warm-Up ____

Strength Training

Exercise		Set 1	Set 2	Set 3	Set 4	Set 5	Set 6
	Reps						
	Weight						
	Reps						
	Weight						
	Reps						
	Weight						
	Reps						
	Weight						
	Reps						
	Weight						
	Reps						
	Weight						
	Reps						
	Weight						
	Reps						
	Weight						
	Reps						
	Weight						

Cardio

Exercise	Calories	Distance	Time

Water Intake ________________

Cooldown ________________

Feeling ☆ ☆ ☆ ☆ ☆

Notes

Today's Goal ____________________   Ⓜ Ⓣ Ⓦ Ⓣ Ⓕ Ⓢ Ⓢ

Muscle Group Focus ____________________   Weight ________   Date/Time __________

Stretch ◯   Warm-Up ____

Strength Training

Exercise		Set 1	Set 2	Set 3	Set 4	Set 5	Set 6
	Reps						
	Weight						
	Reps						
	Weight						
	Reps						
	Weight						
	Reps						
	Weight						
	Reps						
	Weight						
	Reps						
	Weight						
	Reps						
	Weight						
	Reps						
	Weight						
	Reps						
	Weight						
	Reps						
	Weight						

Cardio

Exercise	Calories	Distance	Time

Water Intake ________________________

Cooldown ________________________

Feeling ☆ ☆ ☆ ☆ ☆

Notes

Today's Goal

Today's Goal ________________________ (M) (T) (W) (T) (F) (S) (S)

Muscle Group Focus ________________   Weight ________   Date/Time ________

Stretch ◯   Warm-Up ________________________

Strength Training

Exercise		Set 1	Set 2	Set 3	Set 4	Set 5	Set 6
	Reps						
	Weight						
	Reps						
	Weight						
	Reps						
	Weight						
	Reps						
	Weight						
	Reps						
	Weight						
	Reps						
	Weight						
	Reps						
	Weight						
	Reps						
	Weight						
	Reps						
	Weight						
	Reps						
	Weight						

Cardio

Exercise	Calories	Distance	Time

Water Intake ________________

Cooldown ________________

Feeling ☆ ☆ ☆ ☆ ☆

Notes

Today's Goal ________________ Ⓜ Ⓣ Ⓦ Ⓣ Ⓕ ⬤S ⬤S

Muscle Group Focus ________________ Weight ________ Date/Time ________

Stretch ◯   Warm-Up ________________________________

Strength Training

Exercise		Set 1	Set 2	Set 3	Set 4	Set 5	Set 6
	Reps						
	Weight						
	Reps						
	Weight						
	Reps						
	Weight						
	Reps						
	Weight						
	Reps						
	Weight						
	Reps						
	Weight						
	Reps						
	Weight						
	Reps						
	Weight						
	Reps						
	Weight						
	Reps						
	Weight						

Cardio

Exercise	Calories	Distance	Time

Water Intake ________________

Cooldown ________________

Feeling ☆ ☆ ☆ ☆ ☆

Notes

Today's Goal _______________   (M) (T) (W) (T) (F) (S) (S)

Muscle Group Focus _______________   Weight ________   Date/Time __________

Stretch ◯   Warm-Up _______________________________

Strength Training

Exercise		Set 1	Set 2	Set 3	Set 4	Set 5	Set 6
	Reps						
	Weight						
	Reps						
	Weight						
	Reps						
	Weight						
	Reps						
	Weight						
	Reps						
	Weight						
	Reps						
	Weight						
	Reps						
	Weight						
	Reps						
	Weight						
	Reps						
	Weight						

Cardio

Exercise	Calories	Distance	Time

Water Intake _______________

Cooldown _______________

Feeling ☆ ☆ ☆ ☆ ☆

Notes

Today's Goal _______________________ M T W T F S S

Muscle Group Focus _______________ Weight _______ Date/Time _______

Stretch ◯ Warm-Up _______________________________

Strength Training

Exercise		Set 1	Set 2	Set 3	Set 4	Set 5	Set 6
	Reps						
	Weight						
	Reps						
	Weight						
	Reps						
	Weight						
	Reps						
	Weight						
	Reps						
	Weight						
	Reps						
	Weight						
	Reps						
	Weight						
	Reps						
	Weight						
	Reps						
	Weight						

Cardio

Exercise	Calories	Distance	Time

Water Intake _______________

Cooldown _______________

Feeling ☆ ☆ ☆ ☆ ☆

Notes

Today's Goal ____________________   Ⓜ Ⓣ Ⓦ Ⓣ Ⓕ ⬤S ⬤S

Muscle Group Focus ____________________   Weight ________   Date/Time __________

Stretch ◯   Warm-Up ____

Strength Training

Exercise		Set 1	Set 2	Set 3	Set 4	Set 5	Set 6
	Reps						
	Weight						
	Reps						
	Weight						
	Reps						
	Weight						
	Reps						
	Weight						
	Reps						
	Weight						
	Reps						
	Weight						
	Reps						
	Weight						
	Reps						
	Weight						

Cardio

Exercise	Calories	Distance	Time

Water Intake ____________________

Cooldown ____________________

Feeling ☆ ☆ ☆ ☆ ☆

Notes

Today's Goal   ____________________________   (M) (T) (W) (T) (F) (S) (S)

Muscle Group Focus ____________________   Weight ________   Date/Time _________

Stretch ◯   Warm-Up ____

Strength Training

Exercise		Set 1	Set 2	Set 3	Set 4	Set 5	Set 6
	Reps						
	Weight						
	Reps						
	Weight						
	Reps						
	Weight						
	Reps						
	Weight						
	Reps						
	Weight						
	Reps						
	Weight						
	Reps						
	Weight						
	Reps						
	Weight						
	Reps						
	Weight						
	Reps						
	Weight						

Cardio

Exercise	Calories	Distance	Time

Water Intake _________________

Cooldown _________________

Feeling ☆ ☆ ☆ ☆ ☆

Notes

Today's Goal ________________   (M)(T)(W)(T)(F)(**S**)(**S**)

Muscle Group Focus ________________   Weight _______   Date/Time _______

Stretch ◯   Warm-Up ________________________________

Strength Training

Exercise		Set 1	Set 2	Set 3	Set 4	Set 5	Set 6
	Reps						
	Weight						
	Reps						
	Weight						
	Reps						
	Weight						
	Reps						
	Weight						
	Reps						
	Weight						
	Reps						
	Weight						
	Reps						
	Weight						
	Reps						
	Weight						
	Reps						
	Weight						

Cardio

Exercise	Calories	Distance	Time

Water Intake ________________

Cooldown ________________

Feeling ☆ ☆ ☆ ☆ ☆

Notes

Today's Goal ______________________ Ⓜ Ⓣ Ⓦ Ⓣ Ⓕ ⬤S ⬤S

Muscle Group Focus ______________ Weight ______ Date/Time ________

Stretch ◯ Warm-Up ________________________________

Strength Training

Exercise		Set 1	Set 2	Set 3	Set 4	Set 5	Set 6
	Reps						
	Weight						
	Reps						
	Weight						
	Reps						
	Weight						
	Reps						
	Weight						
	Reps						
	Weight						
	Reps						
	Weight						
	Reps						
	Weight						
	Reps						
	Weight						
	Reps						
	Weight						

Cardio

Exercise	Calories	Distance	Time

Water Intake ________________

Cooldown ________________

Feeling ☆ ☆ ☆ ☆ ☆

Notes

Today's Goal ______________ (M) (T) (W) (T) (F) (S) (S)

Muscle Group Focus ______________ Weight ______ Date/Time ______

Stretch ◯   Warm-Up ______________

Strength Training

Exercise		Set 1	Set 2	Set 3	Set 4	Set 5	Set 6
	Reps						
	Weight						
	Reps						
	Weight						
	Reps						
	Weight						
	Reps						
	Weight						
	Reps						
	Weight						
	Reps						
	Weight						
	Reps						
	Weight						
	Reps						
	Weight						
	Reps						
	Weight						
	Reps						
	Weight						

Cardio

Exercise	Calories	Distance	Time

Water Intake ______________

Cooldown ______________

Feeling ☆ ☆ ☆ ☆ ☆

Notes

Today's Goal

Today's Goal _______________________   (M) (T) (W) (T) (F) (S) (S)

Muscle Group Focus _______________   Weight _______   Date/Time _______

Stretch ◯   Warm-Up _______________________________________

Strength Training

Exercise		Set 1	Set 2	Set 3	Set 4	Set 5	Set 6
	Reps						
	Weight						
	Reps						
	Weight						
	Reps						
	Weight						
	Reps						
	Weight						
	Reps						
	Weight						
	Reps						
	Weight						
	Reps						
	Weight						
	Reps						
	Weight						
	Reps						
	Weight						
	Reps						
	Weight						

Cardio

Exercise	Calories	Distance	Time

Water Intake _______________________

Cooldown _______________________

Feeling ☆ ☆ ☆ ☆ ☆

Notes

Today's Goal ____________________   Ⓜ Ⓣ Ⓦ Ⓣ Ⓕ ⬤S ⬤S

Muscle Group Focus ____________________   Weight ________   Date/Time __________

Stretch ◯   Warm-Up ____________________

Strength Training

Exercise		Set 1	Set 2	Set 3	Set 4	Set 5	Set 6
	Reps						
	Weight						
	Reps						
	Weight						
	Reps						
	Weight						
	Reps						
	Weight						
	Reps						
	Weight						
	Reps						
	Weight						
	Reps						
	Weight						
	Reps						
	Weight						
	Reps						
	Weight						
	Reps						
	Weight						

Cardio

Exercise	Calories	Distance	Time

Water Intake ____________________

Cooldown ____________________

Feeling ☆ ☆ ☆ ☆ ☆

Notes

Today's Goal ___________________   Ⓜ Ⓣ Ⓦ Ⓣ Ⓕ ⬤S ⬤S

Muscle Group Focus _______________   Weight _______   Date/Time _______

Stretch ◯   Warm-Up _______________________________

Strength Training

Exercise		Set 1	Set 2	Set 3	Set 4	Set 5	Set 6
	Reps						
	Weight						
	Reps						
	Weight						
	Reps						
	Weight						
	Reps						
	Weight						
	Reps						
	Weight						
	Reps						
	Weight						
	Reps						
	Weight						
	Reps						
	Weight						
	Reps						
	Weight						

Cardio

Exercise	Calories	Distance	Time

Water Intake _______________

Cooldown _______________

Feeling ☆ ☆ ☆ ☆ ☆

Notes

Today's Goal ______________________

(M) (T) (W) (T) (F) (S) (S)

Muscle Group Focus ______________ Weight ______ Date/Time ______

Stretch ◯ Warm-Up ________________________

Strength Training

Exercise		Set 1	Set 2	Set 3	Set 4	Set 5	Set 6
	Reps						
	Weight						
	Reps						
	Weight						
	Reps						
	Weight						
	Reps						
	Weight						
	Reps						
	Weight						
	Reps						
	Weight						
	Reps						
	Weight						
	Reps						
	Weight						
	Reps						
	Weight						

Cardio

Exercise	Calories	Distance	Time

Water Intake ______________

Cooldown ______________

Feeling ☆ ☆ ☆ ☆ ☆

Notes

Today's Goal ____________________   M T W T F **S** **S**

Muscle Group Focus ____________________   Weight ________   Date/Time ________

Stretch ◯   Warm-Up ____________________

Strength Training

Exercise		Set 1	Set 2	Set 3	Set 4	Set 5	Set 6
	Reps						
	Weight						
	Reps						
	Weight						
	Reps						
	Weight						
	Reps						
	Weight						
	Reps						
	Weight						
	Reps						
	Weight						
	Reps						
	Weight						
	Reps						
	Weight						
	Reps						
	Weight						
	Reps						
	Weight						

Cardio

Exercise	Calories	Distance	Time

Water Intake ____________________

Cooldown ____________________

Feeling ☆ ☆ ☆ ☆ ☆

Notes

Today's Goal ________________________ Ⓜ Ⓣ Ⓦ Ⓣ Ⓕ ⬤S ⬤S

Muscle Group Focus ________________   Weight _______   Date/Time __________

Stretch ◯   Warm-Up ____

Strength Training

Exercise		Set 1	Set 2	Set 3	Set 4	Set 5	Set 6
	Reps						
	Weight						
	Reps						
	Weight						
	Reps						
	Weight						
	Reps						
	Weight						
	Reps						
	Weight						
	Reps						
	Weight						
	Reps						
	Weight						
	Reps						
	Weight						
	Reps						
	Weight						

Cardio

Exercise	Calories	Distance	Time

Water Intake ________________

Cooldown ________________

Feeling ☆ ☆ ☆ ☆ ☆

Notes

Today's Goal ______________________   (M) (T) (W) (T) (F) (S) (S)

Muscle Group Focus ______________   Weight ________   Date/Time __________

Stretch ◯   Warm-Up ________________________________

Strength Training

Exercise		Set 1	Set 2	Set 3	Set 4	Set 5	Set 6
	Reps						
	Weight						
	Reps						
	Weight						
	Reps						
	Weight						
	Reps						
	Weight						
	Reps						
	Weight						
	Reps						
	Weight						
	Reps						
	Weight						
	Reps						
	Weight						
	Reps						
	Weight						
	Reps						
	Weight						

Cardio

Exercise	Calories	Distance	Time

Water Intake ________________

Cooldown ________________

Feeling ☆ ☆ ☆ ☆ ☆

Notes

Today's Goal

(M) (T) (W) (T) (F) **(S)** **(S)**

Muscle Group Focus ________________   Weight ________   Date/Time ________

Stretch ◯   Warm-Up ________________________________

Strength Training

Exercise		Set 1	Set 2	Set 3	Set 4	Set 5	Set 6
	Reps						
	Weight						
	Reps						
	Weight						
	Reps						
	Weight						
	Reps						
	Weight						
	Reps						
	Weight						
	Reps						
	Weight						
	Reps						
	Weight						
	Reps						
	Weight						
	Reps						
	Weight						

Cardio

Exercise	Calories	Distance	Time

Water Intake ________________

Cooldown ________________

Feeling ☆ ☆ ☆ ☆ ☆

Notes

Today's Goal ___________________ (M) (T) (W) (T) (F) (S) (S)

Muscle Group Focus ___________________ Weight _______ Date/Time _______

Stretch ◯   Warm-Up ___________________

Strength Training

Exercise		Set 1	Set 2	Set 3	Set 4	Set 5	Set 6
	Reps						
	Weight						
	Reps						
	Weight						
	Reps						
	Weight						
	Reps						
	Weight						
	Reps						
	Weight						
	Reps						
	Weight						
	Reps						
	Weight						
	Reps						
	Weight						
	Reps						
	Weight						
	Reps						
	Weight						

Cardio

Exercise	Calories	Distance	Time

Water Intake ___________________

Cooldown ___________________

Feeling ☆ ☆ ☆ ☆ ☆

Notes

Today's Goal ___________________   Ⓜ Ⓣ Ⓦ Ⓣ Ⓕ **Ⓢ** **Ⓢ**

Muscle Group Focus _____________________   Weight _________   Date/Time __________

Stretch ◯   Warm-Up ____

Strength Training

Exercise		Set 1	Set 2	Set 3	Set 4	Set 5	Set 6
	Reps						
	Weight						
	Reps						
	Weight						
	Reps						
	Weight						
	Reps						
	Weight						
	Reps						
	Weight						
	Reps						
	Weight						
	Reps						
	Weight						
	Reps						
	Weight						
	Reps						
	Weight						
	Reps						
	Weight						

Cardio

Exercise	Calories	Distance	Time

Water Intake __________________

Cooldown __________________

Feeling ☆ ☆ ☆ ☆ ☆

Notes

Today's Goal

M T W T F **S** **S**

Muscle Group Focus ____________ Weight ______ Date/Time ______

Stretch ◯ Warm-Up ____________

Strength Training

Exercise		Set 1	Set 2	Set 3	Set 4	Set 5	Set 6
	Reps						
	Weight						
	Reps						
	Weight						
	Reps						
	Weight						
	Reps						
	Weight						
	Reps						
	Weight						
	Reps						
	Weight						
	Reps						
	Weight						
	Reps						
	Weight						
	Reps						
	Weight						

Cardio

Exercise	Calories	Distance	Time

Water Intake ____________

Cooldown ____________

Feeling ☆ ☆ ☆ ☆ ☆

Notes

Today's Goal ___________________   （M）（T）（W）（T）（F）（S）（S）

Muscle Group Focus _______________   Weight _______   Date/Time _______

Stretch ◯   Warm-Up _______________________________________

Strength Training

Exercise		Set 1	Set 2	Set 3	Set 4	Set 5	Set 6
	Reps						
	Weight						
	Reps						
	Weight						
	Reps						
	Weight						
	Reps						
	Weight						
	Reps						
	Weight						
	Reps						
	Weight						
	Reps						
	Weight						
	Reps						
	Weight						
	Reps						
	Weight						

Cardio

Exercise	Calories	Distance	Time

Water Intake _______________

Cooldown _______________

Feeling ☆ ☆ ☆ ☆ ☆

Notes

Today's Goal ______________________   Ⓜ Ⓣ Ⓦ Ⓣ Ⓕ Ⓢ Ⓢ

Muscle Group Focus ________________   Weight ________   Date/Time __________

Stretch ◯   Warm-Up ________________________________

Strength Training

Exercise		Set 1	Set 2	Set 3	Set 4	Set 5	Set 6
	Reps						
	Weight						
	Reps						
	Weight						
	Reps						
	Weight						
	Reps						
	Weight						
	Reps						
	Weight						
	Reps						
	Weight						
	Reps						
	Weight						
	Reps						
	Weight						
	Reps						
	Weight						
	Reps						
	Weight						

Cardio

Exercise	Calories	Distance	Time

Water Intake ________________

Cooldown ________________

Feeling ☆ ☆ ☆ ☆ ☆

Notes

Today's Goal ________________________   (M) (T) (W) (T) (F) (S) (S)

Muscle Group Focus ____________________   Weight ________   Date/Time ____________

Stretch ◯   Warm-Up ____

Strength Training

Exercise		Set 1	Set 2	Set 3	Set 4	Set 5	Set 6
	Reps						
	Weight						
	Reps						
	Weight						
	Reps						
	Weight						
	Reps						
	Weight						
	Reps						
	Weight						
	Reps						
	Weight						
	Reps						
	Weight						
	Reps						
	Weight						
	Reps						
	Weight						

Cardio

Exercise	Calories	Distance	Time

Water Intake ____________________

Cooldown ____________________

Feeling ☆ ☆ ☆ ☆ ☆

Notes

Today's Goal ___________________ (M)(T)(W)(T)(F)(**S**)(**S**)

Muscle Group Focus ________________   Weight ________   Date/Time __________

Stretch ◯   Warm-Up ____

Strength Training

Exercise		Set 1	Set 2	Set 3	Set 4	Set 5	Set 6
	Reps						
	Weight						
	Reps						
	Weight						
	Reps						
	Weight						
	Reps						
	Weight						
	Reps						
	Weight						
	Reps						
	Weight						
	Reps						
	Weight						
	Reps						
	Weight						
	Reps						
	Weight						
	Reps						
	Weight						

Cardio

Exercise	Calories	Distance	Time

Water Intake ___________________

Cooldown ___________________

Feeling ☆ ☆ ☆ ☆ ☆

Notes

Today's Goal

M T W T F **S** **S**

Muscle Group Focus ______________ Weight ______ Date/Time ______

Stretch ◯   Warm-Up ______________

Strength Training

Exercise		Set 1	Set 2	Set 3	Set 4	Set 5	Set 6
	Reps						
	Weight						
	Reps						
	Weight						
	Reps						
	Weight						
	Reps						
	Weight						
	Reps						
	Weight						
	Reps						
	Weight						
	Reps						
	Weight						
	Reps						
	Weight						

Cardio

Exercise	Calories	Distance	Time

Water Intake ______________

Cooldown ______________

Feeling ☆ ☆ ☆ ☆ ☆

Notes

Today's Goal

M T W T F S S

Muscle Group Focus ___________________   Weight _______   Date/Time _______

Stretch ◯   Warm-Up ________________________________

Strength Training

Exercise		Set 1	Set 2	Set 3	Set 4	Set 5	Set 6
	Reps						
	Weight						
	Reps						
	Weight						
	Reps						
	Weight						
	Reps						
	Weight						
	Reps						
	Weight						
	Reps						
	Weight						
	Reps						
	Weight						
	Reps						
	Weight						
	Reps						
	Weight						
	Reps						
	Weight						

Cardio

Exercise	Calories	Distance	Time

Water Intake ________________

Cooldown ________________

Feeling ☆ ☆ ☆ ☆ ☆

Notes

Today's Goal _______________   Ⓜ Ⓣ Ⓦ Ⓣ Ⓕ ⬤S ⬤S

Muscle Group Focus _______________   Weight _______   Date/Time _______

Stretch ◯   Warm-Up _____________________________________

Strength Training

Exercise		Set 1	Set 2	Set 3	Set 4	Set 5	Set 6
	Reps						
	Weight						
	Reps						
	Weight						
	Reps						
	Weight						
	Reps						
	Weight						
	Reps						
	Weight						
	Reps						
	Weight						
	Reps						
	Weight						
	Reps						
	Weight						
	Reps						
	Weight						
	Reps						
	Weight						

Cardio

Exercise	Calories	Distance	Time

Water Intake _______________

Cooldown _______________

Feeling ☆ ☆ ☆ ☆ ☆

Notes

Today's Goal _____________________

(M) (T) (W) (T) (F) (S) (S)

Muscle Group Focus _____________________   Weight _______   Date/Time _______

Stretch ◯   Warm-Up _____________________

Strength Training

Exercise		Set 1	Set 2	Set 3	Set 4	Set 5	Set 6
	Reps						
	Weight						
	Reps						
	Weight						
	Reps						
	Weight						
	Reps						
	Weight						
	Reps						
	Weight						
	Reps						
	Weight						
	Reps						
	Weight						
	Reps						
	Weight						
	Reps						
	Weight						
	Reps						
	Weight						

Cardio

Exercise	Calories	Distance	Time

Water Intake _____________________

Cooldown _____________________

Feeling ☆ ☆ ☆ ☆ ☆

Notes

Today's Goal

(M) (T) (W) (T) (F) (**S**) (**S**)

Muscle Group Focus ___________________   Weight _________   Date/Time ___________

Stretch ◯   Warm-Up ____

Strength Training

Exercise		Set 1	Set 2	Set 3	Set 4	Set 5	Set 6
	Reps						
	Weight						
	Reps						
	Weight						
	Reps						
	Weight						
	Reps						
	Weight						
	Reps						
	Weight						
	Reps						
	Weight						
	Reps						
	Weight						
	Reps						
	Weight						
	Reps						
	Weight						

Cardio

Exercise	Calories	Distance	Time

Water Intake ___________________

Cooldown ___________________

Feeling ☆ ☆ ☆ ☆ ☆

Notes

Today's Goal ___________________ Ⓜ Ⓣ Ⓦ Ⓣ Ⓕ ⬤S ⬤S

Muscle Group Focus ______________ Weight ______ Date/Time ______

Stretch ◯ Warm-Up ______________________________________

Strength Training

Exercise		Set 1	Set 2	Set 3	Set 4	Set 5	Set 6
	Reps						
	Weight						
	Reps						
	Weight						
	Reps						
	Weight						
	Reps						
	Weight						
	Reps						
	Weight						
	Reps						
	Weight						
	Reps						
	Weight						
	Reps						
	Weight						
	Reps						
	Weight						
	Reps						
	Weight						

Cardio

Exercise	Calories	Distance	Time

Water Intake ______________________

Cooldown ______________________

Feeling ☆ ☆ ☆ ☆ ☆

Notes

Today's Goal ____________________   (M) (T) (W) (T) (F) (S) (S)

Muscle Group Focus ____________________   Weight ________   Date/Time __________

Stretch ◯   Warm-Up ______________________________________

Strength Training

Exercise		Set 1	Set 2	Set 3	Set 4	Set 5	Set 6
	Reps						
	Weight						
	Reps						
	Weight						
	Reps						
	Weight						
	Reps						
	Weight						
	Reps						
	Weight						
	Reps						
	Weight						
	Reps						
	Weight						
	Reps						
	Weight						
	Reps						
	Weight						

Cardio

Exercise	Calories	Distance	Time

Water Intake ______________________

Cooldown ______________________

Feeling ☆ ☆ ☆ ☆ ☆

Notes

Today's Goal

(M) (T) (W) (T) (F) (S) (S)

Muscle Group Focus ___________________ Weight _______ Date/Time _______

Stretch ◯   Warm-Up ___________________________________

Strength Training

Exercise		Set 1	Set 2	Set 3	Set 4	Set 5	Set 6
	Reps						
	Weight						
	Reps						
	Weight						
	Reps						
	Weight						
	Reps						
	Weight						
	Reps						
	Weight						
	Reps						
	Weight						
	Reps						
	Weight						
	Reps						
	Weight						
	Reps						
	Weight						

Cardio

Exercise	Calories	Distance	Time

Water Intake ___________________

Cooldown ___________________

Feeling ☆ ☆ ☆ ☆ ☆

Notes

Today's Goal _______________________ Ⓜ Ⓣ Ⓦ Ⓣ Ⓕ ⬤S ⬤S

Muscle Group Focus ___________________ Weight _______ Date/Time _______

Stretch ◯   Warm-Up ___________________________________

Strength Training

Exercise		Set 1	Set 2	Set 3	Set 4	Set 5	Set 6
	Reps						
	Weight						
	Reps						
	Weight						
	Reps						
	Weight						
	Reps						
	Weight						
	Reps						
	Weight						
	Reps						
	Weight						
	Reps						
	Weight						
	Reps						
	Weight						
	Reps						
	Weight						

Cardio

Exercise	Calories	Distance	Time

Water Intake _______________________

Cooldown _______________________

Feeling ☆ ☆ ☆ ☆ ☆

Notes

Today's Goal ________________________   Ⓜ Ⓣ Ⓦ Ⓣ Ⓕ ⬤S ⬤S

Muscle Group Focus ________________   Weight ________   Date/Time __________

Stretch ◯   Warm-Up ________________________________

Strength Training

Exercise		Set 1	Set 2	Set 3	Set 4	Set 5	Set 6
	Reps						
	Weight						
	Reps						
	Weight						
	Reps						
	Weight						
	Reps						
	Weight						
	Reps						
	Weight						
	Reps						
	Weight						
	Reps						
	Weight						
	Reps						
	Weight						
	Reps						
	Weight						
	Reps						
	Weight						

Cardio

Exercise	Calories	Distance	Time

Water Intake ________________

Cooldown ________________

Feeling ☆ ☆ ☆ ☆ ☆

Notes

Today's Goal ___________________________   (M) (T) (W) (T) (F) (S) (S)

Muscle Group Focus ______________________   Weight _______   Date/Time __________

Stretch ◯   Warm-Up ____

Strength Training

Exercise			Set 1	Set 2	Set 3	Set 4	Set 5	Set 6
		Reps						
		Weight						
		Reps						
		Weight						
		Reps						
		Weight						
		Reps						
		Weight						
		Reps						
		Weight						
		Reps						
		Weight						
		Reps						
		Weight						
		Reps						
		Weight						
		Reps						
		Weight						

Cardio

Exercise	Calories	Distance	Time

Water Intake _______________

Cooldown _______________

Feeling ☆ ☆ ☆ ☆ ☆

Notes

Today's Goal ________________ Ⓜ Ⓣ Ⓦ Ⓣ Ⓕ ⬤S ⬤S

Muscle Group Focus ________________   Weight ________   Date/Time ________

Stretch ◯   Warm-Up ________________________________

Strength Training

Exercise		Set 1	Set 2	Set 3	Set 4	Set 5	Set 6
	Reps						
	Weight						
	Reps						
	Weight						
	Reps						
	Weight						
	Reps						
	Weight						
	Reps						
	Weight						
	Reps						
	Weight						
	Reps						
	Weight						
	Reps						
	Weight						
	Reps						
	Weight						
	Reps						
	Weight						

Cardio

Exercise	Calories	Distance	Time

Water Intake ________________

Cooldown ________________

Feeling ☆ ☆ ☆ ☆ ☆

Notes

Today's Goal ___________________   (M) (T) (W) (T) (F) (S) (S)

Muscle Group Focus ___________________   Weight ________   Date/Time ___________

Stretch ◯   Warm-Up ____

Strength Training

Exercise		Set 1	Set 2	Set 3	Set 4	Set 5	Set 6
	Reps						
	Weight						
	Reps						
	Weight						
	Reps						
	Weight						
	Reps						
	Weight						
	Reps						
	Weight						
	Reps						
	Weight						
	Reps						
	Weight						
	Reps						
	Weight						
	Reps						
	Weight						

Cardio

Exercise		Calories	Distance	Time

Water Intake ___________________

Cooldown ___________________

Feeling ☆ ☆ ☆ ☆ ☆

Notes

Today's Goal _______________ (M) (T) (W) (T) (F) (S) (S)

Muscle Group Focus _______________   Weight _______   Date/Time _______

Stretch ◯   Warm-Up _______________________________

Strength Training

Exercise		Set 1	Set 2	Set 3	Set 4	Set 5	Set 6
	Reps						
	Weight						
	Reps						
	Weight						
	Reps						
	Weight						
	Reps						
	Weight						
	Reps						
	Weight						
	Reps						
	Weight						
	Reps						
	Weight						
	Reps						
	Weight						
	Reps						
	Weight						
	Reps						
	Weight						

Cardio

Exercise	Calories	Distance	Time

Water Intake _______________

Cooldown _______________

Feeling ☆ ☆ ☆ ☆ ☆

Notes

Today's Goal ___________________ (M) (T) (W) (T) (F) (S) (S)

Muscle Group Focus ________________ Weight ________ Date/Time ________

Stretch ◯   Warm-Up ___________________________________

Strength Training

Exercise		Set 1	Set 2	Set 3	Set 4	Set 5	Set 6
	Reps						
	Weight						
	Reps						
	Weight						
	Reps						
	Weight						
	Reps						
	Weight						
	Reps						
	Weight						
	Reps						
	Weight						
	Reps						
	Weight						
	Reps						
	Weight						
	Reps						
	Weight						

Cardio

Exercise	Calories	Distance	Time

Water Intake ____________

Cooldown ____________

Feeling ☆ ☆ ☆ ☆ ☆

Notes

Today's Goal

M T W T F **S** **S**

Muscle Group Focus ___________________ Weight _______ Date/Time _________

Stretch ◯ Warm-Up _______________________________

Strength Training

Exercise		Set 1	Set 2	Set 3	Set 4	Set 5	Set 6
	Reps						
	Weight						
	Reps						
	Weight						
	Reps						
	Weight						
	Reps						
	Weight						
	Reps						
	Weight						
	Reps						
	Weight						
	Reps						
	Weight						
	Reps						
	Weight						
	Reps						
	Weight						

Cardio

Exercise	Calories	Distance	Time

Water Intake _______________

Cooldown _______________

Feeling ☆ ☆ ☆ ☆ ☆

Notes

Today's Goal ______________________   (M) (T) (W) (T) (F) (S) (S)

Muscle Group Focus ______________   Weight ______   Date/Time ______

Stretch ◯   Warm-Up ______________________

Strength Training

Exercise		Set 1	Set 2	Set 3	Set 4	Set 5	Set 6
	Reps						
	Weight						
	Reps						
	Weight						
	Reps						
	Weight						
	Reps						
	Weight						
	Reps						
	Weight						
	Reps						
	Weight						
	Reps						
	Weight						
	Reps						
	Weight						
	Reps						
	Weight						
	Reps						
	Weight						

Cardio

Exercise	Calories	Distance	Time

Water Intake ______________

Cooldown ______________

Feeling ☆ ☆ ☆ ☆ ☆

Notes

Today's Goal ___________________   Ⓜ Ⓣ Ⓦ Ⓣ Ⓕ ⬤S ⬤S

Muscle Group Focus ___________________   Weight _______   Date/Time _________

Stretch ◯   Warm-Up _______________________________________

Strength Training

Exercise		Set 1	Set 2	Set 3	Set 4	Set 5	Set 6
	Reps						
	Weight						
	Reps						
	Weight						
	Reps						
	Weight						
	Reps						
	Weight						
	Reps						
	Weight						
	Reps						
	Weight						
	Reps						
	Weight						
	Reps						
	Weight						
	Reps						
	Weight						

Cardio

Exercise	Calories	Distance	Time

Water Intake _______________________

Cooldown _______________________

Feeling ☆ ☆ ☆ ☆ ☆

Notes

Today's Goal _______________________   (M) (T) (W) (T) (F) (S) (S)

Muscle Group Focus _______________   Weight _______   Date/Time _______

Stretch ◯   Warm-Up _________________________________

Strength Training

Exercise		Set 1	Set 2	Set 3	Set 4	Set 5	Set 6
	Reps						
	Weight						
	Reps						
	Weight						
	Reps						
	Weight						
	Reps						
	Weight						
	Reps						
	Weight						
	Reps						
	Weight						
	Reps						
	Weight						
	Reps						
	Weight						
	Reps						
	Weight						

Cardio

Exercise	Calories	Distance	Time

Water Intake _________________

Cooldown _________________

Feeling ☆ ☆ ☆ ☆ ☆

Notes

Today's Goal ___________ Ⓜ Ⓣ Ⓦ Ⓣ Ⓕ **Ⓢ** **Ⓢ**

Muscle Group Focus ___________   Weight _______   Date/Time _______

Stretch ◯   Warm-Up ___________

Strength Training

Exercise		Set 1	Set 2	Set 3	Set 4	Set 5	Set 6
	Reps						
	Weight						
	Reps						
	Weight						
	Reps						
	Weight						
	Reps						
	Weight						
	Reps						
	Weight						
	Reps						
	Weight						
	Reps						
	Weight						
	Reps						
	Weight						
	Reps						
	Weight						

Cardio

Exercise	Calories	Distance	Time

Water Intake ___________

Cooldown ___________

Feeling ☆ ☆ ☆ ☆ ☆

Notes

Today's Goal ___________________   (M) (T) (W) (T) (F) (S) (S)

Muscle Group Focus ___________________   Weight _______   Date/Time _________

Stretch ◯   Warm-Up ___________________________________

Strength Training

Exercise		Set 1	Set 2	Set 3	Set 4	Set 5	Set 6
	Reps						
	Weight						
	Reps						
	Weight						
	Reps						
	Weight						
	Reps						
	Weight						
	Reps						
	Weight						
	Reps						
	Weight						
	Reps						
	Weight						
	Reps						
	Weight						
	Reps						
	Weight						
	Reps						
	Weight						

Cardio

Exercise	Calories	Distance	Time

Water Intake ___________________

Cooldown ___________________

Feeling ☆ ☆ ☆ ☆ ☆

Notes

Today's Goal ____________________   (M) (T) (W) (T) (F) (S) (S)

Muscle Group Focus ________________   Weight ______   Date/Time __________

Stretch ◯   Warm-Up ____

Strength Training

Exercise		Set 1	Set 2	Set 3	Set 4	Set 5	Set 6
	Reps						
	Weight						
	Reps						
	Weight						
	Reps						
	Weight						
	Reps						
	Weight						
	Reps						
	Weight						
	Reps						
	Weight						
	Reps						
	Weight						
	Reps						
	Weight						
	Reps						
	Weight						
	Reps						
	Weight						

Cardio

Exercise	Calories	Distance	Time

Water Intake ____________________

Cooldown ____________________

Feeling ☆ ☆ ☆ ☆ ☆

Notes

Today's Goal ____________________   (M) (T) (W) (T) (F) (S) (S)

Muscle Group Focus ________________   Weight ________   Date/Time ________

Stretch ◯   Warm-Up ____

Strength Training

Exercise		Set 1	Set 2	Set 3	Set 4	Set 5	Set 6
	Reps						
	Weight						
	Reps						
	Weight						
	Reps						
	Weight						
	Reps						
	Weight						
	Reps						
	Weight						
	Reps						
	Weight						
	Reps						
	Weight						
	Reps						
	Weight						
	Reps						
	Weight						
	Reps						
	Weight						

Cardio

Exercise	Calories	Distance	Time

Water Intake ________________

Cooldown ________________

Feeling ☆ ☆ ☆ ☆ ☆

Notes

Today's Goal __________________________   Ⓜ Ⓣ Ⓦ Ⓣ Ⓕ Ⓢ Ⓢ

Muscle Group Focus __________________   Weight ________   Date/Time __________

Stretch ◯   Warm-Up ____

Strength Training

Exercise		Set 1	Set 2	Set 3	Set 4	Set 5	Set 6
	Reps						
	Weight						
	Reps						
	Weight						
	Reps						
	Weight						
	Reps						
	Weight						
	Reps						
	Weight						
	Reps						
	Weight						
	Reps						
	Weight						
	Reps						
	Weight						
	Reps						
	Weight						

Cardio

Exercise	Calories	Distance	Time

Water Intake __________________

Cooldown __________________

Feeling ☆ ☆ ☆ ☆ ☆

Notes

Today's Goal

(M) (T) (W) (T) (F) (S) (S)

Muscle Group Focus ____________________ Weight ________ Date/Time ____________

Stretch ◯   Warm-Up ________________________________

Strength Training

Exercise		Set 1	Set 2	Set 3	Set 4	Set 5	Set 6
	Reps						
	Weight						
	Reps						
	Weight						
	Reps						
	Weight						
	Reps						
	Weight						
	Reps						
	Weight						
	Reps						
	Weight						
	Reps						
	Weight						
	Reps						
	Weight						
	Reps						
	Weight						

Cardio

Exercise	Calories	Distance	Time

Water Intake ____________________

Cooldown ____________________

Feeling ☆ ☆ ☆ ☆ ☆

Notes

Today's Goal   __________________   (M) (T) (W) (T) (F) **(S)** **(S)**

Muscle Group Focus ________________   Weight ________   Date/Time ________

Stretch ◯   Warm-Up ____

Strength Training

Exercise		Set 1	Set 2	Set 3	Set 4	Set 5	Set 6
	Reps						
	Weight						
	Reps						
	Weight						
	Reps						
	Weight						
	Reps						
	Weight						
	Reps						
	Weight						
	Reps						
	Weight						
	Reps						
	Weight						
	Reps						
	Weight						
	Reps						
	Weight						
	Reps						
	Weight						

Cardio

Exercise	Calories	Distance	Time

Water Intake ________________

Cooldown ________________

Feeling ☆ ☆ ☆ ☆ ☆

Notes

Today's Goal _______________________ Ⓜ Ⓣ Ⓦ Ⓣ Ⓕ ⬤S ⬤S

Muscle Group Focus _______________ Weight _______ Date/Time _______

Stretch ◯   Warm-Up _______________________________

Strength Training

Exercise		Set 1	Set 2	Set 3	Set 4	Set 5	Set 6
	Reps						
	Weight						
	Reps						
	Weight						
	Reps						
	Weight						
	Reps						
	Weight						
	Reps						
	Weight						
	Reps						
	Weight						
	Reps						
	Weight						
	Reps						
	Weight						
	Reps						
	Weight						

Cardio

Exercise	Calories	Distance	Time

Water Intake _______________

Cooldown _______________

Feeling ☆ ☆ ☆ ☆ ☆

Notes

Today's Goal ___________ Ⓜ Ⓣ Ⓦ Ⓣ Ⓕ ⬤S ⬤S

Muscle Group Focus _____________ Weight ______ Date/Time ________

Stretch ◯   Warm-Up ____________________________

Strength Training

Exercise		Set 1	Set 2	Set 3	Set 4	Set 5	Set 6
	Reps						
	Weight						
	Reps						
	Weight						
	Reps						
	Weight						
	Reps						
	Weight						
	Reps						
	Weight						
	Reps						
	Weight						
	Reps						
	Weight						
	Reps						
	Weight						
	Reps						
	Weight						
	Reps						
	Weight						

Cardio

Exercise	Calories	Distance	Time

Water Intake ________________

Cooldown ________________

Feeling ☆ ☆ ☆ ☆ ☆

Notes

Today's Goal _________________________ Ⓜ Ⓣ Ⓦ Ⓣ Ⓕ ⬤S ⬤S

Muscle Group Focus _________________ Weight ________ Date/Time _________

Stretch ◯   Warm-Up _________________________________

Strength Training

Exercise		Set 1	Set 2	Set 3	Set 4	Set 5	Set 6
	Reps						
	Weight						
	Reps						
	Weight						
	Reps						
	Weight						
	Reps						
	Weight						
	Reps						
	Weight						
	Reps						
	Weight						
	Reps						
	Weight						
	Reps						
	Weight						
	Reps						
	Weight						

Cardio

Exercise	Calories	Distance	Time

Water Intake _________________

Cooldown _________________

Feeling ☆ ☆ ☆ ☆ ☆

Notes

Today's Goal ____________________ Ⓜ Ⓣ Ⓦ Ⓣ Ⓕ ⚫S ⚫S

Muscle Group Focus ____________________ Weight ________ Date/Time ____________

Stretch ◯ Warm-Up ____

Strength Training

Exercise		Set 1	Set 2	Set 3	Set 4	Set 5	Set 6
	Reps						
	Weight						
	Reps						
	Weight						
	Reps						
	Weight						
	Reps						
	Weight						
	Reps						
	Weight						
	Reps						
	Weight						
	Reps						
	Weight						
	Reps						
	Weight						
	Reps						
	Weight						
	Reps						
	Weight						

Cardio

Exercise	Calories	Distance	Time

Water Intake ____________________

Cooldown ____________________

Feeling ☆ ☆ ☆ ☆ ☆

Notes

Today's Goal __________________   (M) (T) (W) (T) (F) **(S)** **(S)**

Muscle Group Focus __________________   Weight ________   Date/Time __________

Stretch ◯   Warm-Up __________________________________

Strength Training

Exercise		Set 1	Set 2	Set 3	Set 4	Set 5	Set 6
	Reps						
	Weight						
	Reps						
	Weight						
	Reps						
	Weight						
	Reps						
	Weight						
	Reps						
	Weight						
	Reps						
	Weight						
	Reps						
	Weight						
	Reps						
	Weight						

Cardio

Exercise	Calories	Distance	Time

Water Intake __________________

Cooldown __________________

Feeling ☆ ☆ ☆ ☆ ☆

Notes

Today's Goal _______________   Ⓜ Ⓣ Ⓦ Ⓣ Ⓕ ⑤ ⑤

Muscle Group Focus _______________   Weight _______   Date/Time _______

Stretch ◯   Warm-Up _______________________________

Strength Training

Exercise		Set 1	Set 2	Set 3	Set 4	Set 5	Set 6
	Reps						
	Weight						
	Reps						
	Weight						
	Reps						
	Weight						
	Reps						
	Weight						
	Reps						
	Weight						
	Reps						
	Weight						
	Reps						
	Weight						
	Reps						
	Weight						
	Reps						
	Weight						

Cardio

Exercise	Calories	Distance	Time

Water Intake _______________

Cooldown _______________

Feeling ☆ ☆ ☆ ☆ ☆

Notes

Today's Goal ____________________   (M) (T) (W) (T) (F) (S) (S)

Muscle Group Focus ____________________   Weight ________   Date/Time __________

Stretch ◯   Warm-Up ____

Strength Training

Exercise		Set 1	Set 2	Set 3	Set 4	Set 5	Set 6
	Reps						
	Weight						
	Reps						
	Weight						
	Reps						
	Weight						
	Reps						
	Weight						
	Reps						
	Weight						
	Reps						
	Weight						
	Reps						
	Weight						
	Reps						
	Weight						
	Reps						
	Weight						
	Reps						
	Weight						

Cardio

Exercise	Calories	Distance	Time

Water Intake ________________

Cooldown ________________

Feeling ☆ ☆ ☆ ☆ ☆

Notes

Today's Goal ___________________ (M) (T) (W) (T) (F) (S) (S)

Muscle Group Focus ___________________ Weight _______ Date/Time __________

Stretch ◯   Warm-Up ____

Strength Training

Exercise		Set 1	Set 2	Set 3	Set 4	Set 5	Set 6
	Reps						
	Weight						
	Reps						
	Weight						
	Reps						
	Weight						
	Reps						
	Weight						
	Reps						
	Weight						
	Reps						
	Weight						
	Reps						
	Weight						
	Reps						
	Weight						
	Reps						
	Weight						

Cardio

Exercise	Calories	Distance	Time

Water Intake ___________________

Cooldown ___________________

Feeling ☆ ☆ ☆ ☆ ☆

Notes

Today's Goal ___________________ (M) (T) (W) (T) (F) (S) (S)

Muscle Group Focus _______________   Weight ________   Date/Time __________

Stretch ◯   Warm-Up _______________________________________

Strength Training

Exercise		Set 1	Set 2	Set 3	Set 4	Set 5	Set 6
	Reps						
	Weight						
	Reps						
	Weight						
	Reps						
	Weight						
	Reps						
	Weight						
	Reps						
	Weight						
	Reps						
	Weight						
	Reps						
	Weight						
	Reps						
	Weight						
	Reps						
	Weight						
	Reps						
	Weight						

Cardio

Exercise	Calories	Distance	Time

Water Intake _______________

Cooldown _______________

Feeling ☆ ☆ ☆ ☆ ☆

Notes

Today's Goal ___________________ (M) (T) (W) (T) (F) **(S)** **(S)**

Muscle Group Focus _______________ Weight _______ Date/Time _________

Stretch ◯   Warm-Up _______________________________

Strength Training

Exercise		Set 1	Set 2	Set 3	Set 4	Set 5	Set 6
	Reps						
	Weight						
	Reps						
	Weight						
	Reps						
	Weight						
	Reps						
	Weight						
	Reps						
	Weight						
	Reps						
	Weight						
	Reps						
	Weight						
	Reps						
	Weight						
	Reps						
	Weight						
	Reps						
	Weight						

Cardio

Exercise	Calories	Distance	Time

Water Intake _______________

Cooldown _______________

Feeling ☆ ☆ ☆ ☆ ☆

Notes

Today's Goal

M T W T F S S

Muscle Group Focus _______________ Weight _______ Date/Time _______

Stretch ◯   Warm-Up _______________________

Strength Training

Exercise		Set 1	Set 2	Set 3	Set 4	Set 5	Set 6
	Reps						
	Weight						
	Reps						
	Weight						
	Reps						
	Weight						
	Reps						
	Weight						
	Reps						
	Weight						
	Reps						
	Weight						
	Reps						
	Weight						
	Reps						
	Weight						
	Reps						
	Weight						

Cardio

Exercise	Calories	Distance	Time

Water Intake _______________

Cooldown _______________

Feeling ☆ ☆ ☆ ☆ ☆

Notes

Today's Goal _______________ Ⓜ Ⓣ Ⓦ Ⓣ Ⓕ ⚫S ⚫S

Muscle Group Focus _______________ Weight _______ Date/Time _______

Stretch ◯   Warm-Up _________________________________

Strength Training

Exercise		Set 1	Set 2	Set 3	Set 4	Set 5	Set 6
	Reps						
	Weight						
	Reps						
	Weight						
	Reps						
	Weight						
	Reps						
	Weight						
	Reps						
	Weight						
	Reps						
	Weight						
	Reps						
	Weight						
	Reps						
	Weight						
	Reps						
	Weight						
	Reps						
	Weight						

Cardio

Exercise	Calories	Distance	Time

Water Intake _________________

Cooldown _________________

Feeling ☆ ☆ ☆ ☆ ☆

Notes

Today's Goal   (M) (T) (W) (T) (F) (S) (S)

Muscle Group Focus ____________________   Weight ______   Date/Time ________

Stretch ◯   Warm-Up ________________________________

Strength Training

Exercise		Set 1	Set 2	Set 3	Set 4	Set 5	Set 6
	Reps						
	Weight						
	Reps						
	Weight						
	Reps						
	Weight						
	Reps						
	Weight						
	Reps						
	Weight						
	Reps						
	Weight						
	Reps						
	Weight						
	Reps						
	Weight						
	Reps						
	Weight						

Cardio

Exercise	Calories	Distance	Time

Water Intake ________________

Cooldown ________________

Feeling ☆ ☆ ☆ ☆ ☆

Notes

Today's Goal ___________________   (M) (T) (W) (T) (F) (S) (S)

Muscle Group Focus ___________________   Weight _______   Date/Time ___________

Stretch ◯   Warm-Up ____

Strength Training

Exercise		Set 1	Set 2	Set 3	Set 4	Set 5	Set 6
	Reps						
	Weight						
	Reps						
	Weight						
	Reps						
	Weight						
	Reps						
	Weight						
	Reps						
	Weight						
	Reps						
	Weight						
	Reps						
	Weight						
	Reps						
	Weight						
	Reps						
	Weight						

Cardio

Exercise	Calories	Distance	Time

Water Intake ___________________

Cooldown ___________________

Feeling ☆ ☆ ☆ ☆ ☆

Notes

Today's Goal ______________________ M T W T F **S** **S**

Muscle Group Focus ______________ Weight ______ Date/Time ______

Stretch ○   Warm-Up ____

Strength Training

Exercise		Set 1	Set 2	Set 3	Set 4	Set 5	Set 6
	Reps						
	Weight						
	Reps						
	Weight						
	Reps						
	Weight						
	Reps						
	Weight						
	Reps						
	Weight						
	Reps						
	Weight						
	Reps						
	Weight						
	Reps						
	Weight						
	Reps						
	Weight						
	Reps						
	Weight						

Cardio

Exercise	Calories	Distance	Time

Water Intake ______________

Cooldown ______________

Feeling ☆ ☆ ☆ ☆ ☆

Notes

Today's Goal ___________________ M T W T F S S

Muscle Group Focus ___________________ Weight ________ Date/Time __________

Stretch ◯ Warm-Up ___________________

Strength Training

Exercise		Set 1	Set 2	Set 3	Set 4	Set 5	Set 6
	Reps						
	Weight						
	Reps						
	Weight						
	Reps						
	Weight						
	Reps						
	Weight						
	Reps						
	Weight						
	Reps						
	Weight						
	Reps						
	Weight						
	Reps						
	Weight						
	Reps						
	Weight						

Cardio

Exercise	Calories	Distance	Time

Water Intake ___________________

Cooldown ___________________

Feeling ☆ ☆ ☆ ☆ ☆

Notes

Today's Goal ______________________   (M) (T) (W) (T) (F) (S) (S)

Muscle Group Focus ______________   Weight ________   Date/Time ________

Stretch ◯   Warm-Up ______________________________________

Strength Training

Exercise		Set 1	Set 2	Set 3	Set 4	Set 5	Set 6
	Reps						
	Weight						
	Reps						
	Weight						
	Reps						
	Weight						
	Reps						
	Weight						
	Reps						
	Weight						
	Reps						
	Weight						
	Reps						
	Weight						
	Reps						
	Weight						
	Reps						
	Weight						

Cardio

Exercise	Calories	Distance	Time

Water Intake ______________

Cooldown ______________

Feeling ☆ ☆ ☆ ☆ ☆

Notes

Today's Goal ______________________   Ⓜ Ⓣ Ⓦ Ⓣ Ⓕ ⚫S ⚫S

Muscle Group Focus ______________   Weight ______   Date/Time __________

Stretch ◯   Warm-Up ____

Strength Training

Exercise		Set 1	Set 2	Set 3	Set 4	Set 5	Set 6
	Reps						
	Weight						
	Reps						
	Weight						
	Reps						
	Weight						
	Reps						
	Weight						
	Reps						
	Weight						
	Reps						
	Weight						
	Reps						
	Weight						
	Reps						
	Weight						
	Reps						
	Weight						
	Reps						
	Weight						

Cardio

Exercise	Calories	Distance	Time

Water Intake ________________

Cooldown ________________

Feeling ☆ ☆ ☆ ☆ ☆

Notes

Today's Goal ______________ M T W T F S S

Muscle Group Focus ______________   Weight ________   Date/Time ________

Stretch ◯   Warm-Up ______________

Strength Training

Exercise		Set 1	Set 2	Set 3	Set 4	Set 5	Set 6
	Reps						
	Weight						
	Reps						
	Weight						
	Reps						
	Weight						
	Reps						
	Weight						
	Reps						
	Weight						
	Reps						
	Weight						
	Reps						
	Weight						
	Reps						
	Weight						
	Reps						
	Weight						
	Reps						
	Weight						

Cardio

Exercise	Calories	Distance	Time

Water Intake ______________

Cooldown ______________

Feeling ☆ ☆ ☆ ☆ ☆

Notes

Today's Goal _______________ Ⓜ Ⓣ Ⓦ Ⓣ Ⓕ Ⓢ Ⓢ

Muscle Group Focus _______________ Weight _______ Date/Time _______

Stretch ◯   Warm-Up _______________________________

Strength Training

Exercise		Set 1	Set 2	Set 3	Set 4	Set 5	Set 6
	Reps						
	Weight						
	Reps						
	Weight						
	Reps						
	Weight						
	Reps						
	Weight						
	Reps						
	Weight						
	Reps						
	Weight						
	Reps						
	Weight						
	Reps						
	Weight						
	Reps						
	Weight						
	Reps						
	Weight						

Cardio

Exercise	Calories	Distance	Time

Water Intake _______________

Cooldown _______________

Feeling ☆ ☆ ☆ ☆ ☆

Notes

Today's Goal

(M) (T) (W) (T) (F) (**S**) (**S**)

Muscle Group Focus ______________________   Weight ________   Date/Time __________

Stretch ◯   Warm-Up ____

Strength Training

Exercise		Set 1	Set 2	Set 3	Set 4	Set 5	Set 6
	Reps						
	Weight						
	Reps						
	Weight						
	Reps						
	Weight						
	Reps						
	Weight						
	Reps						
	Weight						
	Reps						
	Weight						
	Reps						
	Weight						
	Reps						
	Weight						
	Reps						
	Weight						

Cardio

Exercise	Calories	Distance	Time

Water Intake ________________

Cooldown ________________

Feeling ☆ ☆ ☆ ☆ ☆

Notes

Today's Goal

M T W T F **S** **S**

Muscle Group Focus ___________ Weight _______ Date/Time _______

Stretch ◯ Warm-Up _______________________

Strength Training

Exercise		Set 1	Set 2	Set 3	Set 4	Set 5	Set 6
	Reps						
	Weight						
	Reps						
	Weight						
	Reps						
	Weight						
	Reps						
	Weight						
	Reps						
	Weight						
	Reps						
	Weight						
	Reps						
	Weight						
	Reps						
	Weight						
	Reps						
	Weight						

Cardio

Exercise	Calories	Distance	Time

Water Intake _______________

Cooldown _______________

Feeling ☆ ☆ ☆ ☆ ☆

Notes

Today's Goal _______________________   Ⓜ Ⓣ Ⓦ Ⓣ Ⓕ ⬤S ⬤S

Muscle Group Focus _______________   Weight _______   Date/Time _______

Stretch ◯   Warm-Up _______________________

Strength Training

Exercise		Set 1	Set 2	Set 3	Set 4	Set 5	Set 6
	Reps						
	Weight						
	Reps						
	Weight						
	Reps						
	Weight						
	Reps						
	Weight						
	Reps						
	Weight						
	Reps						
	Weight						
	Reps						
	Weight						
	Reps						
	Weight						
	Reps						
	Weight						

Cardio

Exercise	Calories	Distance	Time

Water Intake _______________

Cooldown _______________

Feeling ☆ ☆ ☆ ☆ ☆

Notes

Today's Goal _______________ Ⓜ Ⓣ Ⓦ Ⓣ Ⓕ Ⓢ Ⓢ

Muscle Group Focus _______________   Weight _______   Date/Time _______

Stretch ◯   Warm-Up _______________

Strength Training

Exercise		Set 1	Set 2	Set 3	Set 4	Set 5	Set 6
	Reps						
	Weight						
	Reps						
	Weight						
	Reps						
	Weight						
	Reps						
	Weight						
	Reps						
	Weight						
	Reps						
	Weight						
	Reps						
	Weight						
	Reps						
	Weight						
	Reps						
	Weight						
	Reps						
	Weight						

Cardio

Exercise	Calories	Distance	Time

Water Intake _______________

Cooldown _______________

Feeling ☆ ☆ ☆ ☆ ☆

Notes

Today's Goal __________________________   Ⓜ Ⓣ Ⓦ Ⓣ Ⓕ ⬤S ⬤S

Muscle Group Focus __________________   Weight _______   Date/Time _________

Stretch ◯   Warm-Up ____

Strength Training

Exercise		Set 1	Set 2	Set 3	Set 4	Set 5	Set 6
	Reps						
	Weight						
	Reps						
	Weight						
	Reps						
	Weight						
	Reps						
	Weight						
	Reps						
	Weight						
	Reps						
	Weight						
	Reps						
	Weight						
	Reps						
	Weight						
	Reps						
	Weight						
	Reps						
	Weight						

Cardio

Exercise	Calories	Distance	Time

Water Intake _______________________

Cooldown _________________________

Feeling ☆ ☆ ☆ ☆ ☆

Notes

Today's Goal ______________________   Ⓜ Ⓣ Ⓦ Ⓣ Ⓕ ⚫ ⚫

Muscle Group Focus ______________   Weight ______   Date/Time ________

Stretch ◯   Warm-Up ________________________________

Strength Training

Exercise		Set 1	Set 2	Set 3	Set 4	Set 5	Set 6
	Reps						
	Weight						
	Reps						
	Weight						
	Reps						
	Weight						
	Reps						
	Weight						
	Reps						
	Weight						
	Reps						
	Weight						
	Reps						
	Weight						
	Reps						
	Weight						
	Reps						
	Weight						
	Reps						
	Weight						

Cardio

Exercise	Calories	Distance	Time

Water Intake ________________

Cooldown ________________

Feeling ☆ ☆ ☆ ☆ ☆

Notes

Today's Goal   ________________   Ⓜ Ⓣ Ⓦ Ⓣ Ⓕ ⬤S ⬤S

Muscle Group Focus ________________   Weight ________   Date/Time ________

Stretch ◯   Warm-Up ________________________________

Strength Training

Exercise		Set 1	Set 2	Set 3	Set 4	Set 5	Set 6
	Reps						
	Weight						
	Reps						
	Weight						
	Reps						
	Weight						
	Reps						
	Weight						
	Reps						
	Weight						
	Reps						
	Weight						
	Reps						
	Weight						
	Reps						
	Weight						
	Reps						
	Weight						
	Reps						
	Weight						

Cardio

Exercise	Calories	Distance	Time

Water Intake ________________

Cooldown ________________

Feeling ☆ ☆ ☆ ☆ ☆

Notes

Today's Goal _______________ Ⓜ Ⓣ Ⓦ Ⓣ Ⓕ Ⓢ Ⓢ

Muscle Group Focus _______________   Weight _______   Date/Time _______

Stretch ◯   Warm-Up _______________

Strength Training

Exercise		Set 1	Set 2	Set 3	Set 4	Set 5	Set 6
	Reps						
	Weight						
	Reps						
	Weight						
	Reps						
	Weight						
	Reps						
	Weight						
	Reps						
	Weight						
	Reps						
	Weight						
	Reps						
	Weight						
	Reps						
	Weight						
	Reps						
	Weight						
	Reps						
	Weight						

Cardio

Exercise	Calories	Distance	Time

Water Intake _______________

Cooldown _______________

Feeling ☆ ☆ ☆ ☆ ☆

Notes

Today's Goal _______________   Ⓜ Ⓣ Ⓦ Ⓣ Ⓕ ⬤S ⬤S

Muscle Group Focus _______________   Weight _______   Date/Time _______

Stretch ◯   Warm-Up _______________

Strength Training

Exercise		Set 1	Set 2	Set 3	Set 4	Set 5	Set 6
	Reps						
	Weight						
	Reps						
	Weight						
	Reps						
	Weight						
	Reps						
	Weight						
	Reps						
	Weight						
	Reps						
	Weight						
	Reps						
	Weight						
	Reps						
	Weight						
	Reps						
	Weight						
	Reps						
	Weight						

Cardio

Exercise	Calories	Distance	Time

Water Intake _______________

Cooldown _______________

Feeling ☆ ☆ ☆ ☆ ☆

Notes

Today's Goal ____________________   Ⓜ Ⓣ Ⓦ Ⓣ Ⓕ ⬤S ⬤S

Muscle Group Focus ____________________   Weight ________   Date/Time __________

Stretch ◯   Warm-Up ____________________

Strength Training

Exercise		Set 1	Set 2	Set 3	Set 4	Set 5	Set 6
	Reps						
	Weight						
	Reps						
	Weight						
	Reps						
	Weight						
	Reps						
	Weight						
	Reps						
	Weight						
	Reps						
	Weight						
	Reps						
	Weight						
	Reps						
	Weight						
	Reps						
	Weight						

Cardio

Exercise	Calories	Distance	Time

Water Intake ____________________

Cooldown ____________________

Feeling ☆ ☆ ☆ ☆ ☆

Notes

Today's Goal _______________   (M) (T) (W) (T) (F) (S) (S)

Muscle Group Focus _______________   Weight _______   Date/Time _______

Stretch ◯   Warm-Up _______________

Strength Training

Exercise		Set 1	Set 2	Set 3	Set 4	Set 5	Set 6
	Reps						
	Weight						
	Reps						
	Weight						
	Reps						
	Weight						
	Reps						
	Weight						
	Reps						
	Weight						
	Reps						
	Weight						
	Reps						
	Weight						
	Reps						
	Weight						
	Reps						
	Weight						

Cardio

Exercise	Calories	Distance	Time

Water Intake _______________

Cooldown _______________

Feeling ☆ ☆ ☆ ☆ ☆

Notes

www.ingramcontent.com/pod-product-compliance
Lightning Source LLC
Chambersburg PA
CBHW081304250726

48662CB00008B/2386